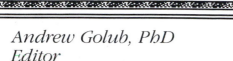

*Andrew Golub, PhD*
*Editor*

# The Cultural/Subcultural Contexts of Marijuana Use at the Turn of the Twenty-First Century

*The Cultural/Subcultural Contexts of Marijuana Use at the Turn of the Twenty-First Century has been co-published simultaneously as Journal of Ethnicity in Substance Abuse, Volume 4, Numbers 3/4 2005.*

*Pre-publication REVIEWS, COMMENTARIES, EVALUATIONS . . .*

"This book ILLUMINATES CORNERS OF THE MARIJUANA CONTROVERSY RARELY MENTIONED IN THE PRESS OR BY PUBLIC OFFICIALS. Instead of stereotypical 'druggies,' stumbling aimlessly through a 'gateway' toward addiction and despair, we meet a variety of rational, sensible, and moderate marijuana users in a variety of settings, from gritty urban neighborhoods to comfortable, white suburbs. What these marijuana users have in common is a remarkable similarity to social drinkers, with their marijuana use governed by both spoken and unspoken rules that discourage excess, and which seem to be based on thoroughly reasonable risk/benefit assessments. Policymakers, who often seem to pretend that such people do not exist, would do well to try to understand them instead."

**Bruce Mirken**
*Director of Communications*
*Marijuana Policy Project*

"Anyone wishing to understand the diverse cultures of marijuana users in the US in the new century should consider this book REQUIRED READING. Dr. Golub's presentation of the epidemiology of marijuana use is followed by a set of chapters filled with rich descriptions of everything from the role of blunts in the resurgence of marijuana use, to its use by gang members in San Francisco, adults in Oklahoma City, and even by medical marijuana dispensing organizations in California."

**Eric D. Wish, PhD**
*Director*
*Center for Substance Abuse Research (CESAR)*
*University of Maryland*

The Haworth Press, Inc.

# The Cultural/Subcultural Contexts of Marijuana Use at the Turn of the Twenty-First Century

*The Cultural/Subcultural Contexts of Marijuana Use at the Turn of the Twenty-First Century* has been co-published simultaneously as *Journal of Ethnicity in Substance Abuse,* Volume 4, Numbers 3/4 2005.

## Monographic Separates from the *Journal of Ethnicity in Substance Abuse*™

For additional information on these and other Haworth Press titles, including descriptions, tables of contents, reviews, and prices, use the QuickSearch catalog at http://www.HaworthPress.com.

The *Journal of Ethnicity in Substance Abuse*™ is the successor title to *Drugs & Society,* which changed title after Vol. 16, No. 1/2 2000. The journal is renumbered to start as Vol. 1, No. 1 2002.

***The Cultural/Subcultural Contexts of Marijuana Use at the Turn of the Twenty-First Century,*** edited by Andrew Golub, PhD (Vol. 4, No. 3/4, 2005). "*TIMELY. . . . Relies on both quantitative and qualitative data sources to provide AN EXCELLENT OVERVIEW OF CURRENT TRENDS. Readers will benefit overall from the extensive coverage of the current cultural and subcultural forms of marijuana use. While appealing to a wide audience of academic and policymakers this book should also prove interesting to members of the general public who are concerned about the social problem of illicit drug use*" (Margaret S. Kelley, PhD, Assistant Professor, Department of Sociology, University of Oklahoma)

***New Drugs on the Street: Changing Inner City Patterns of Illicit Consumption,*** edited by Merrill Singer, PhD (Vol. 4, No. 2, 2005). "*ESSENTIAL READING for anyone in the drug use area who wants to be brought up-to-date on the current state of the field. This edited work provides an excellent look at a number of emerging drug use trends. This includes new drugs appearing in particular areas, drugs appearing among different subpopulations, and gaining a better understanding of the composition of drugs already being used.*" (Scott Clair, PhD, Associate Scientist, Partnerships in Prevention Science Institute, Iowa State University)

# The Cultural/Subcultural Contexts of Marijuana Use at the Turn of the Twenty-First Century

Andrew Golub, PhD
Editor

*The Cultural/Subcultural Contexts of Marijuana Use at the Turn of the Twenty-First Century* has been co-published simultaneously as *Journal of Ethnicity in Substance Abuse*, Volume 4, Numbers 3/4 2005.

The Haworth Press, Inc.

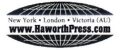

New York • London • Victoria (AU)
www.HaworthPress.com

*The Cultural/Subcultural Contexts of Marijuana Use at the Turn of the Twenty-First Century* has been co-published simultaneously as *Journal of Ethnicity in Substance Abuse*™, Volume 4, Numbers 3/4 2005.

The development, preparation, and publication of this work has been undertaken with great care. However, the publisher, employees, editors, and agents of The Haworth Press and all imprints of The Haworth Press, Inc., including The Haworth Medical Press® and Pharmaceutical Products Press®, are not responsible for any errors contained herein or for consequences that may ensue from use of materials or information contained in this work. With regard to case studies, identities and circumstances of individuals discussed herein have been changed to protect confidentiality. Any resemblance to actual persons, living or dead, is entirely coincidental.

The Haworth Press is committed to the dissemination of ideas and information according to the highest standards of intellectual freedom and the free exchange of ideas. Statements made and opinions expressed in this publication do not necessarily reflect the views of the Publisher, Directors, management, or staff of The Haworth Press, Inc., or an endorsement by them.

Cover design by Kerry Mack
Cover photos:
"Caselined," by Flutura Bardhi
"Bong," by Flutura Bardhi
"Bluntroll," by Anthony Nguyen
"Cruiser," by Anthony Nguyen

**Library of Congress Cataloging-in-Publication Data**

Cataloging-in-Publication Data
The cultural/subcultural contexts of marijuana use at the turn of the twenty-first century/Andrew Golub
    p. cm
        "Co-published simultaneously as Journal of Ethnicity in Substance Abuse, Volume 4, Numbers 3/4."
        Includes bibliographical references and index.
        ISBN-13: 978-0-7890-3203-4 (hard cover: alk. paper)
        ISBN-10: 0-7890-3203-1 (hard cover: alk. paper)
        ISBN-13: 978-0-7890-3204-1 (soft cover: alk. paper)
        ISBN-10: 0-7890-3204-X (soft cover: alk. paper)
        1. Marijuana–Social aspects. 2. Marijuana in popular culture. 3. Marijuana abuse. I. Golub, Andrew Lang. II. Journal of ethnicity in substance abuse.
HV5822.M3C784 2005
306´.1–dc22
        2005031513

# Indexing, Abstracting & Website/Internet Coverage

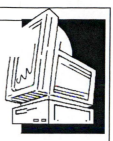

This section provides you with a list of major indexing & abstracting services and other tools for bibliographic access. That is to say, each service began covering this periodical during the year noted in the right column. Most Websites which are listed below have indicated that they will either post, disseminate, compile, archive, cite or alert their own Website users with research-based content from this work. (This list is as current as the copyright date of this publication.)

Abstracting, Website/Indexing Coverage . . . . . . . . . Year When Coverage Began

- *Abstracts in Anthropology*
  *<http://www.baywood.com/Journals/PreviewJournals.asp?
  Id=0001-3455>* . . . . . . . . . . . . . . . . . . . . . . . . . . . . . . . . . . . **1991**

- *Academic Abstracts/CD-ROM* . . . . . . . . . . . . . . . . . . . . . . . . **1995**

- *Academic Search Elite (EBSCO)* . . . . . . . . . . . . . . . . . . . . . . **1993**

- *Addiction Abstracts is a quarterly journal published in simultaneous
  print & online editions. This unique resource & reference tool
  is published in collaboration with the Nat'l Addiction Ctr &
  Carfax, Taylor & Francis.
  <http://www.tandf.co.uk/addiction-abs>* . . . . . . . . . . . . . . . . . . **1994**

- *Applied Social Sciences Index & Abstracts (ASSIA)
  (Online: ASSI via Data-Star) (CDRom: ASSIA Plus)
  <http://www.csa.com>* . . . . . . . . . . . . . . . . . . . . . . . . . . . . . . . **1987**

- *Business Source Corporate: coverage of nearly 3,350 quality
  magazines and journals; designed to meet the diverse
  information needs of corporations; EBSCO Publishing
  <http://www.epnet.com/corporate/bsourcecorp.asp>* . . . . . . . . **2002**

- *CAB ABSTRACTS c/o CAB International/CAB ACCESS . . .
  available in print, diskettes updated weekly, and on INTERNET.
  Providing full bibliographic listings, author affiliation,
  augmented keyword searching. <http://www.cabi.org/>* . . . . . **2004**

(continued)

(continued)

(continued)

(continued)

  **\*Exact start date to come.**

*Special Bibliographic Notes related to special journal issues (separates) and indexing/abstracting:*

- indexing/abstracting services in this list will also cover material in any "separate" that is co-published simultaneously with Haworth's special thematic journal issue or DocuSerial. Indexing/abstracting usually covers material at the article/chapter level.
- monographic co-editions are intended for either non-subscribers or libraries which intend to purchase a second copy for their circulating collections.
- monographic co-editions are reported to all jobbers/wholesalers/approval plans. The source journal is listed as the "series" to assist the prevention of duplicate purchasing in the same manner utilized for books-in-series.
- to facilitate user/access services all indexing/abstracting services are encouraged to utilize the co-indexing entry note indicated at the bottom of the first page of each article/chapter/contribution.
- this is intended to assist a library user of any reference tool (whether print, electronic, online, or CD-ROM) to locate the monographic version if the library has purchased this version but not a subscription to the source journal.
- individual articles/chapters in any Haworth publication are also available through the Haworth Document Delivery Service (HDDS).

# The Cultural/Subcultural Contexts of Marijuana Use at the Turn of the Twenty-First Century

## CONTENTS

# ABOUT THE EDITOR

**Andrew Golub, PhD,** is Principal Investigator at National Development and Research Institutes [NDRI], Inc. He also teaches Drugs and Society at the University of Vermont. He holds a PhD in Public Policy Analysis from Carnegie Mellon University. His research focuses on understanding social conditions with an aim towards developing appropriate public policies. Much of his work has focused on understanding the ebb and flow in the popularity of various illicit drugs as recorded in statistics and based in personal and social experiences.

# The Growth in Marijuana Use Among American Youths During the 1990s and the Extent of Blunt Smoking

Andrew Golub, PhD
Bruce D. Johnson, PhD
Eloise Dunlap, PhD

**SUMMARY.** Marijuana use among American youths and young adults increased substantially during the 1990s. This paper reviews that trend using data collected 1979-2003 by the National Survey on Drug Use and Health (NSDUH). The data suggest that the increase in marijuana use started first among persons age 12-20. Among 18-20 year-olds, the increase started earlier among whites and blacks than Hispanics, among males before females, and surprisingly in areas that are not part of an MSA as opposed to those with a population in excess of a million.

Much of the increase in marijuana use could have been attributable to

Andrew Golub is Principal Investigator, and Bruce D. Johnson and Eloise Dunlap are affiliated with the National Development and Research Institutes [NDRI], Inc.

Address correspondence to: Andrew Golub, PhD, National Development & Research Institutes, 71 West 23rd Street, 8th Floor, New York, NY 10010 (E-mail: andrewgolub@verizon.net).

The analyses presented were supported by a grant from the National Institute on Drug Abuse (R01 DA13690-04 and R01 DA09056-03).

Points of view and opinions expressed do not necessarily reflect the positions of the National Institute on Drug Abuse nor National Development and Research Institutes.

[Haworth co-indexing entry note]: "The Growth in Marijuana Use Among American Youths During the 1990s and the Extent of Blunt Smoking." Golub, Andrew, Bruce D. Johnson, and Eloise Dunlap. Co-published simultaneously in *Journal of Ethnicity in Substance Abuse* (The Haworth Press, Inc.) Vol. 4, No. 3/4, 2005, pp. 1-21; and: *The Cultural/Subcultural Contexts of Marijuana Use at the Turn of the Twenty-First Century* (ed: Andrew Golub ) The Haworth Press, Inc., 2005, pp. 1-21. Single or multiple copies of this article are available for a fee from The Haworth Document Delivery Service [1-800-HAWORTH, 9:00 a.m. - 5:00 p.m. (EST). E-mail address: docdelivery@haworthpress.com].

*1*

the growing popularity of blunts. Starting in 2000, the NSDUH explicitly asked youths age 12-17 (but not older respondents) about smoking blunts. Of the 9% of youths who reported past-30-day use of marijuana 2000-03, more than half reported smoking blunts. On the other hand, the data also indicate that blunts have not fully supplanted other ways that youths consume marijuana. Blunts were more common among youths that were black, older, male, and from metropolitan areas. Many blunt smokers reported they had not used marijuana, which suggests that they did not define smoking blunts as marijuana use. Even fewer reported that they had used cigars, suggesting they did not define smoking blunts as cigar use. *[Article copies available for a fee from The Haworth Document Delivery Service: 1-800-HAWORTH. E-mail address: <docdelivery@haworthpress.com> Website: <http://www.HaworthPress.com> © 2005 by The Haworth Press, Inc. All rights reserved.]*

**KEYWORDS.** Marijuana, blunts, drug eras, youth

## *INTRODUCTION*

During the 1990s, the use of marijuana increased substantially, especially among youths (Gfroerer, Wu & Penne, 2002; Golub & Johnson, 2001; Golub et al., 2004; Johnston, O'Malley, & Bachman, 2003). This paper reviews this finding using data collected by the National Survey on Drug Use and Health (NSDUH, formerly the National Household Survey on Drug Abuse or NHSDA) from 1979 to 2003 and explores the extent to which this increase may have been associated with the growing popularity of blunts using data collected by the NSDUH from 2000 to 2003.

### *A Conceptual Model of a Drug Era*

The interpretation of marijuana use trends was guided by our conceptual model for the natural course of a drug era (see Golub, Johnson, & Dunlap, 2005). Based on empirical and theoretical research, we conceptualize four distinct phases to drug eras: incubation, expansion, plateau and decline. This framework has been previously used to analyze the Heroin Injection Era prevailing in the 1960s and early 1970s (Golub & Johnson, 2005; Johnson & Golub, 2002), the Crack Era of the late 1980s and early 1990s (Golub & Johnson, 1997), the Marijuana/Blunts Era of the 1990s (Golub & Johnson, 1999, 2001; Golub et al., 2004; Johnson, Golub, & Dunlap, 2000), and a modest rise in use of hallucinogens such as MDMA in the 1990s (Golub et al., 2001).

A drug era typically starts among a highly limited subpopulation participating in a specific social context (*incubation phase*). The Marijuana/Blunts Era was based in the hip-hop movement (Sifaneck et al., 2003). Sometimes, the pioneering drug users successfully introduce the practice to wider subgroups of users and to the broader population (*expansion phase*). When ideas spread, they tend to spread with increasing rapidity (Alwin & McCammon, 2003; Rogers, 1995). Eventually, everyone most at risk of the new drug practice (typically users of other illicit drugs) has either initiated use or at least had the opportunity to do so. For a time, widespread use prevails (*plateau phase*). During this period, youths typically initiate use of the currently popular drug(s), if any. These users form the core of a drug generation for whom the drug has particularly symbolic significance based in their social activities and relationships (see Alwin & McCammon, 2003). Eventually, the use of an illicit drug tends to go out of favor (*decline phase*). During the decline phase, a decreasing proportion of youths coming of age develop into users. However, the overall use of the drug endures for many years as some members of a drug generation continue their habits.

## The Role of Blunt Smoking in the Latest Marijuana Era

A few scattered bits of qualitative research and journalistic references suggested that much of the recent increase in marijuana use may have involved smoking blunts, an inexpensive cigar in which the tobacco filler is replaced with marijuana (Boehlert, 1994; Community Epidemiology Work Group 1999; Sifaneck et al., 2003; Yerger, Pearson, & Malone, 2001). References to blunts regularly appeared in rap music, music videos showed rappers and others smoking cigars (presumably blunts), and T-shirts sporting the Phillies Blunt logo sold widely among youths (Sifaneck et al., 2003). The collection of evidence suggested that an interest in smoking blunts and their symbolic importance to youth subculture could be associated with the increase in marijuana use during the 1990s. Until recently, explicit information about the prevalence of blunt smoking was unavailable. During the 1990s, major drug surveys asked about the use of marijuana but not specifically about the use of blunts; this included the NSDUH (Substance Abuse and Mental Health Services Administration, SAMHSA,

2002a) and Monitoring the Future (MTF) (Johnston, Bachman, & O'Malley, 1999).

Estimates for marijuana use may have been biased downward to the extent that youths did not define blunt smoking as marijuana use. The authors of this paper regard blunt smoking as use of marijuana because marijuana is the primary psychoactive substance in a blunt. On the other hand, smoking a blunt does not as clearly constitute cigar use because most of the cigar contents are discarded in preparing a blunt. Yerger et al. (2001) examined youths perceptions of the word "cigar." In 1999, they held six focus groups with 50 African Americans youths age 14-18 in the San Francisco area. They found that youths were confused about whether the term cigar applied to use of small cigars like "Black and Mild" and blunts. One participant said, "When I hear *cigar*, I think old people with them big ones." In 2001, Soldz, Huyser, and Dorsey (2003) explicitly tested whether 5,016 Massachusetts students in grades 7-12 defined blunt smoking as cigar use. They were interested in determining whether increases in youthful cigar use during the 1990s might have been caused by blunt smokers reporting their behavior as cigar smoking. Early in their questionnaire, they asked, "Have you ever smoked a cigar, cigarillo, or little cigar?" Subsequent sections asked about use of blunts and cigars. The cigar use section started with the explanation, "The next questions ask about cigar use. THEY DO NOT INCLUDE BLUNTS" (emphases in original). They found strong agreement (95%) between responses to the two lifetime cigar use questions and concluded that the increase in youthful cigar use during the 1990s was not simply an artifact of blunt smoking being reported as cigar use. Their study also provided some of the most explicit evidence that blunt smoking is quite widespread among youths; 20% reported lifetime use and 10% reported past-30-day use. They found higher rates of blunt smoking among older students and males.

In 2000, the NSDUH introduced several questions regarding the use of blunts that were asked only of respondents age 12-17. Primary reports from the NSDUH program have not yet reported on the use of blunts (Gfroerer et al., 2002; SAMHSA, 2001, 2002b, 2003c). This paper examines responses to questions about smoking blunts as well as use of marijuana and cigars to identify (1) the extent to which youthful marijuana use nationwide involves smoking blunts and the covariates of use; (2) the extent to which youths define blunt smoking as marijuana use; and (3) the extent to which youths define blunt smoking as cigar use.

# METHODS

## The National Survey on Drug Use and Health

The NSDUH was designed to "serve as the primary source of information on the prevalence and incidence of illicit drugs, alcohol, and tobacco use in the civilian non-institutionalized population aged 12 or older in the United States" and has been conducted since 1971 (SAMHSA, 2003a, p. 1). The survey was conducted in 1971 and 1972 and then every two or three years until 1990 when it became an annual survey. The marijuana trend analyses presented in this report are based on the 512,169 responses available in public use data files for surveys conducted in 1979, 1982, 1985, 1988, and 1990-2003.

Various factors can potentially affect the drug use trends measured with the NSDUH including the following (Biemer et al., 1991; Del Bocca & Noll, 2000): sampling plans exclude groups of persons; individuals decline to participate; non-disclosure; distortions to responses; changes in survey procedures across years; and others. These imperfections are less of a problem for analysis of trends to the extent that the characteristics of the survey remained constant over time. However, the NSDUH program has clearly evolved over time. When examining findings, it is important to evaluate whether programmatic changes can potentially account for differences recorded across years.

From 1979 through 1990, the NSDUH sampled non-institutionalized household members in the 48 contiguous states (SAMHSA, 2003b). Starting in 1991, the target population was expanded to include all 50 states and residents of non-institutional group quarters (e.g., college dormitories, group homes, military installations). Persons with no fixed residence, residents of institutions (e.g., jails and hospitals), and active military personnel were still excluded from the sampling frame. In 1994, a dramatically revised questionnaire and new procedures for logical editing of responses were introduced (SAMHSA, 1996). A split sample procedure was employed to test the impact of the redesign. Many of the estimates obtained using the old and new procedures were quite similar–within two percentage points of each other. Generally, estimates obtained using the new instrument were higher for alcohol and tobacco use but lower for illicit drugs.

In 1999, the survey was greatly expanded in order to support state-level estimates of drug use (Gfroerer, Eyerman, & Chromy, 2002). Computer-assisted personal interviewing (CAPI), in which the interviewer records responses in a computer, was introduced for less sensitive information. Audio computer-assisted self-interviewing (ACASI), in which the respondent listens to recorded questions and enters their responses into a computer, was introduced to increase the level of accurate disclosure of illicit drug use and other sensitive behaviors. Prior to 1999, respondents would privately record their responses to alcohol and drug questions on separate sheets not visible to the interviewer.

The NSDUH employs hierarchical stratified sampling to select a representative sample of eligible participants. The NSDUH datafiles include sample weights and respondent strata to account for the complex sampling procedure. Sample weights were used in all calculation presented in this paper to yield unbiased estimates. However, conventional tests of statistical significance that do not account for design effects were used. Typically, clustered samples yield less reliable estimates. Because of such design effects and because of the large number of cases in the sample, the $\alpha = .01$ level was used in all tests of statistical significance. Sample sizes reported represent unweighted counts.

### Analysis of Blunt Smoking

The analysis of blunt smoking was based on information collected 2000-03 from 72,772 respondents age 12-17 (see SAMHSA, 2001, 2002b, 2003c). The NSDUH questions regarding marijuana use mentioned a variety of common techniques for consuming marijuana but did not explicitly mention blunts (SAMHSA, 2002c, pp. 73-76):

> The next questions are about marijuana and hashish. Marijuana is also called pot or grass. Marijuana is usually smoked, either in cigarettes, called joints, or in a pipe. It is sometimes cooked in food. Hashish is a form of marijuana that is also called "hash." It is usually smoked in a pipe. Another form of hashish is hash oil. Have you ever, even once, used marijuana or hashish? . . . During the past 30 days . . .? What is your best estimate of the number of days . . .?

Conceivably, blunt smokers that did not know that blunts contain marijuana may have reported they had not used marijuana. Even blunt smokers aware of the contents may have interpreted the marijuana use question as limited to marijuana consumed alone as in joints or pipes.

The NSDUH questions on blunts explicitly indicated that a blunt contains marijuana. However, the blunt questions appeared after the marijuana questions–too late to possibly clarify for the interviewee whether smoking a blunt constitutes marijuana use (SAMHSA, 2002c, p. 440):

> Sometimes people take some tobacco out of a cigar and replace it with marijuana. This is called a "blunt" or sometimes a "blob." Have you ever smoked part or all of a cigar with marijuana in it? During the past 30 days . . .? On how many of the past 30 days . . .?

A similar lack of explicit guidance potentially affected the interpretation of the NSDUH cigar questions. The following cigar questions appeared before the blunt questions and did not identify whether smoking a blunt constituted cigar use (SAMHSA, 2002c, pp. 60-62):

> The next questions are about smoking cigars. By cigars we mean any kind, including big cigars, cigarillos, and even little cigars that look like cigarettes. Have you ever smoked part or all of any type of cigar? . . . During the past 30 days . . .?

The percentage of blunt smokers among past-30-day marijuana users was estimated as follows:

$$\frac{\text{Number of respondents that smoked a blunt in past 30 days}}{\text{Number of respondents that used marijuana or blunts in past 30 days}} \times 100\%$$

An analogous formula was used for prevalence among lifetime marijuana users. The denominator included all respondents that reported use of either marijuana, blunts, or both (hereafter marijuana/blunts). Some respondents reported use of blunts but not marijuana. These cases could possibly represent individuals that did not define blunt smoking as marijuana use. In fact, this calculation may provide an underestimate. Youths that smoke both blunts and marijuana in other forms (such as joints) will report smoking both blunts and marijuana, even if they do not define smoking blunts as marijuana use.

Three logistic regression models were estimated to examine whether the covariates of marijuana and marijuana/blunt use differed, and to identify which marijuana/blunt users were more likely to use blunts. The first model examined the extent to which past-30-day marijuana use varied with standard demographic variables: age, race/ethnicity, gender, MSA size, and interview year. The second model examined the covariates of marijuana/blunt use. Differences between these models suggested the extent to which estimates for covariates of marijuana use may have been distorted by not explicitly asking about blunts. The last model examined which marijuana/blunt users were more likely to have smoked blunts. Respondents that did not use marijuana/blunts in the past-30-days were excluded from this analysis. For each model, the Wald statistic was used to identify which covariates were statistically significant and as a rough indication of their relative importance (Hosmer & Lemeshow, 1989).

## FINDINGS

### Trends in Marijuana Use

Figure 1 indicates the trends in marijuana use over time and by age group. Back in 1979, the overall prevalence of marijuana use within the general population was 13%. The variation with age followed an inverted U-shaped curve with a peak rate among 18-20 year-olds (40% in 1979) followed by 21-25 year-olds (33%). Rates were substantially lower among older (6% among those age 26+) and younger respondents (17% among those age 12-17). During the 1980s, marijuana use declined overall and within each age category. During the 1990s, the overall rate of marijuana use was about 5%. The decreasing marijuana use in the 1980s represents a decline phase to the widespread popularity of marijuana that prevailed during the 1960s and 1970s that we refer to as the marijuana/joints era to distinguish it from the current period of increased marijuana use.

In 1993, marijuana use started to increase among persons age 12-20. Among 18-20 year-olds, marijuana use increased from 11% in 1992 to 17% in 1996. A similar time trend prevailed among 12-17 year-olds, although the prevalence of marijuana use was lower in each year. Of note, the prevalence among respondents age 21-25 and age 26+ remained generally stable throughout the 1990s. From 1996 to 2000, the prevalence of marijuana use among 12-17 and 18-20 year-olds leveled off at about 8% and 18%, respectively. Based on NSDUH data through 1999, the authors had previously interpreted this stability as suggesting the marijuana upsurge had reached a plateau by 1996 (Golub & Johnson, 2001; Golub et al., 2004). This paper extends that analysis by incorporating four additional years of data continuing through 2003. The designation of a plateau phase in the 2000s is partially supported by a stable rate of marijuana use of 8% among youths age 12-17. However, use had

FIGURE 1. Variation Over Time in Past-30-Day Marijuana Use by AGE, NSDUH 1979-2003

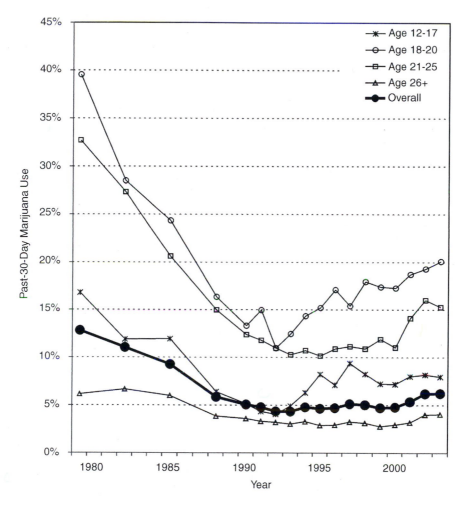

not yet reached peak levels among older age groups: among 18-20 year olds, marijuana use increased from 17% in 2000 up to 20% in 2003; among 21-25 year olds, prevalence jumped from 11% in 2000 to 16% in 2002; and among respondents age 26+ the prevalence increased modestly from 3% in 2000 to 4% in 2003. These increases would appear to represent an aging of the marijuana/blunts generation. Thus, based on the NSDUH data extending through 2003 we generally concur with our previous conclusion that the marijuana/blunts era entered a plateau around 1996 and that by 2003 the era was still in a plateau phase.

The use of blunts was reputedly centered among black males from the inner-city, especially those involved in the New York Hip Hop scene. Golub and Johnson (2001) examined location specific data regarding marijuana use among arrestees across the U.S. Surprisingly, that analysis revealed that the growth in marijuana use started among arrestees in about 1992 in all regions of the country. The following figures use the NSDUH data to examine the extent to which the growth in marijuana use among 18-20 year olds in the general population started earlier among blacks (Figure 2), males (Figure 3) or in metropolitan areas (Figure 4).

The prevalence of marijuana use increased 7 percentage points from 1992 to 1996 among both white and black 18-20 year olds (Figure 2). During the 1990s, white young adults were always a few percentage points more likely to have used marijuana than were blacks. This disparity increased in the 2000s, as the prevalence among white young adults increased from 19% in 2000 to 23% in 2003 but the prevalence among black young adults fluctuated around 15-18%. Thus, the new increase in marijuana use 2000-03 among young adults appears to have been primarily among whites. The increase among Hispanic young adults was not as consistent; a 2 percentage point increase in 1992, and a 4 percentage point increase in 1998. The data indicate that marijuana use is less common among Hispanic young adults and that the marijuana/blunts era may have diffused to this population slightly later than among whites and black.

In 1992, marijuana use was somewhat more common among male young adults (13%) than females (8%). The increase in use started among males in 1993, a year before females. However, both male and female young adults were affected by the increase in marijuana use; by 2003, the prevalence was 24% among males and 16% among females.

There was substantial variation in the timing of the marijuana/blunts era across MSA size, but not in the expected direction (Figure 4).[1] The prevalence of use among young adults in smaller MSAs (with a population of less than 1 million people) varied erratically from 1988 to 1999. We have no clear explanation for why this should be the case. However, as a result it is difficult to definitively identify when the increase in marijuana use started in these areas. Our best guess would be 1993 but perhaps as early 1989. The increase in marijuana use in non-SMA areas appears to have started back in 1991. The increase in larger metropolitan MSAs started in 1993. This was completely unexpected. We have

FIGURE 2. Variation Over Time in Past-30-Day Marijuana Use by RACE/ETHNICITY, NSDUH 1979-2003 Respondents Age 18-20

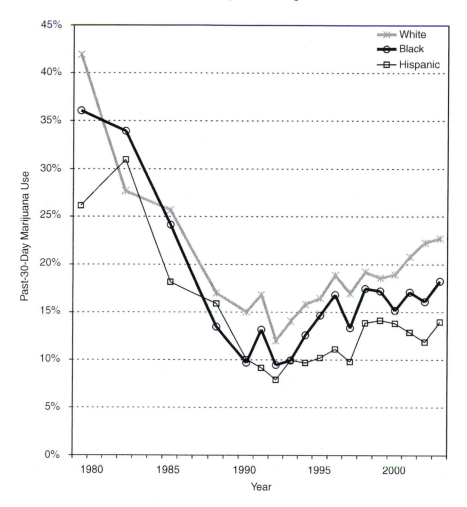

no hypothesis as to why the increase in marijuana use may have started in less densely populated areas before moving to larger MSAs.

### Blunt Smoking Among Youths Age 12-17

Table 1 reports the prevalence of lifetime (21%) and past-30-day (9%) marijuana/blunt use among youths age 12-17. By the 2000s,

FIGURE 3. Variation Over Time in Past-30-Day Marijuana Use by GENDER, NSDUH 1979-2003 Respondents Age 18-20

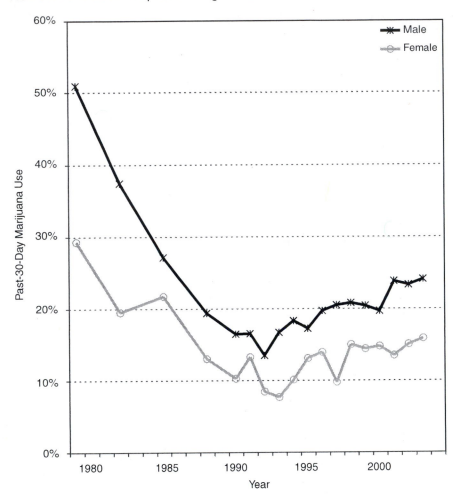

blunts had already become a common method for consuming marijuana; more than half (54-55%) the marijuana/blunt users reported using blunts. Combining the marijuana and blunts responses increased the prevalence of past-30-day use from 8% to 9%, an increase of 16%. An analogous calculation increased the prevalence of lifetime marijuana use by 7%. This suggests that self-reports of marijuana use by 12-17 year olds tend to undercount use because some blunt smokers do not define their behavior as marijuana use.

FIGURE 4. Variation Over Time in Past-30-Day Marijuana Use by MSA SIZE, NSDUH 1979-2003 Respondents Age 18-20

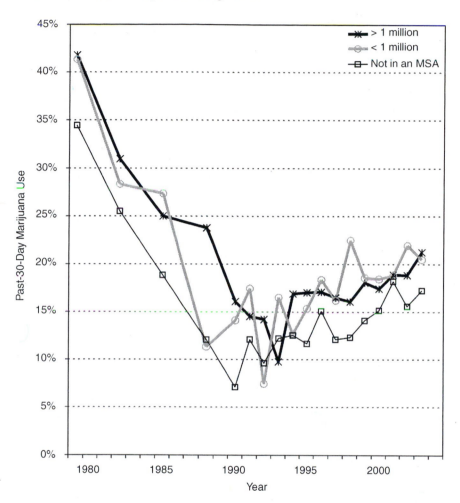

Table 2 examines this definitional issue further. Among past-30-day blunt smokers, more than a quarter (26%) reported they did not smoke marijuana. The reporting rate was lower among lifetime blunt smokers (12%). These estimates of blunt smoking that do not define their behavior as marijuana use are likely to be lower bounds because some youths may have used both blunts and marijuana in other forms, especially

TABLE 1. Prevalence of Marijuana and Blunt Use Among American Youths Age 12-17, NSDUH 2000-2003

|  | Lifetime | Past 30 Days |
|---|---|---|
| (A) Marijuana | 19.6% | 7.8% |
| (B) Blunts | 11.3% | 5.0% |
| (C) Marijuana/blunts (A or B) | 20.9% | 9.1% |
| Increase in marijuana/blunts use over marijuana use (C ÷ A − 1) | 6.9% | 16.1% |
| Blunt use among marijuana/blunt users (B ÷ C) | 53.9% | 54.7% |

TABLE 2. Percentage of Blunt Smokers Who Reported Marijuana and Cigar Use NSDUH Respondents 2000-2003, Age 12-17

|  | Lifetime Blunt Users | Past 30 Day Blunt Users |
|---|---|---|
| Report marijuana use |  |  |
| Yes | 87.6% | 73.5% |
| No | 12.4% | 26.5% |
| Report cigar use |  |  |
| Yes | 59.1% | 32.4% |
| No | 40.9% | 67.6% |

when it comes to questions of lifetime use. The percentage of blunt smokers that define this behavior as cigar use appears to be much lower. Among past-30-day blunt smokers, over two-thirds (68%) reported they had not smoked cigars. Among lifetime blunt smokers, the rate was 41%. Again, these rates are likely to be under-estimates.

The regression models in the first two columns of Table 3 indicate that age was the factor most associated with variation in marijuana and marijuana/blunt use (Wald Statistics of 2,284.4 and 2,570.2).[2] Use of marijuana and marijuana/blunts both increased with age and increased at nearly the same rate for each. The variations associated with age, gender, MSA size and interview year were quite similar for the two models. The modest differences in prevalence rates between whites and blacks

TABLE 3. Covariates of Past-30-Day Marijuana and Blunt Use, NSDUH Respondents 2000-2003, Age 12-17

| | Odds Ratios (Wald Statistics) | | |
| | Marijuana Use | Marijuana/Blunt Use | Blunt Use Given Marijuana/Blunt Use |
|---|---|---|---|
| *Age* | (2,284.4)** | (2,570.2)** | (32.5)** |
| 12 years old | 0.03 | 0.05 | 0.6 |
| 13 years old | 0.1 | 0.1 | 0.8 |
| 14 years old | 0.3 | 0.3 | 0.7 |
| 15 years old | 0.6 | 0.6 | 0.7 |
| 16 years old | 0.8 | 0.8 | 0.9 |
| 17 years old[a] | 1.0 | 1.0 | 1.0 |
| *Race/Ethnicity* | (89.2)** | (152.0)** | (80.8)** |
| White[a] | 1.0 | 1.0 | 1.0 |
| Black | 0.7 | 0.9 | 2.8 |
| Hispanic | 0.8 | 0.9 | 1.2 |
| Other | 0.7 | 0.7 | 1.1 |
| *Gender* | (65.0)** | (76.9)** | (29.2)** |
| .Male[a] | 1.0 | 1.0 | 1.0 |
| Female | 0.8 | 0.8 | 0.8 |
| *MSA Size* | (18.5)** | (26.4)** | (24.3)** |
| Over 1 million[a] | 1.0 | 1.0 | 1.0 |
| Under 1 million | 1.1 | 1.1 | 1.1 |
| Not an MSA | 0.9 | 0.9 | 0.8 |
| *Interview Year* | (17.5)** | (14.4)** | (13.8)** |
| 2000 | 0.9 | 0.9 | 1.1 |
| 2001 | 1.0 | 1.0 | 0.9 |
| 2002 | 1.0 | 1.0 | 1.2 |
| 2003[a] | 1.0 | 1.0 | 1.0 |
| Constant | 0.24 | 0.27 | 1.4 |
| Sample size | 72,772 | 72,430 | 6,750 |

**Wald statistic significant at the $\alpha = .01$ level.
[a]Reference category.

and between whites and Hispanics diminished with the inclusion of blunt use.

The regression analysis of blunt smoking among marijuana/blunt users in the third column of Table 3 indicates the most variation was associated with race/ethnicity (Wald statistic = 152.0). Black youths that smoked marijuana/blunts were substantially more likely to smoke blunts than youths of other race/ethnicities (Odds Ratio = 2.8). The prevalence of blunt use was also somewhat higher for older respondents, males, and youths from metropolitan areas.

Table 4 presents the bivariate variations in marijuana use, marijuana/blunt use, and blunt use among marijuana/blunt users associated with each of the demographic factors considered in Table 3. Marijuana use increased steadily with age from about 1% to over 16%. Marijuana/blunt use was slightly higher than marijuana use at each age reaching more than 18% at age 17. About half the marijuana/blunt users at each age smoked blunts; the rates were slightly higher among 16-17 year olds (56-58%) than among 12-15 year olds (48-52%).

Most blacks (almost three quarters) who used marijuana/blunts smoked blunts, as opposed to about half among whites and Hispanics. Conversely, black blunt smokers may have been less likely to have consumed marijuana in other forms (lower bound of 26%) than white blunt smokers (49%). Moreover, black blunt smokers were more likely to define their activity as not marijuana use than were white blunt smokers. Marijuana/blunt use was 2.4 percentage points higher than marijuana use among black youths (see Table 4). In contrast, the difference for white youths was only 1.1 percentage points. The difference for Hispanic youths (1.4 percentage points) was slightly greater than for white youths but substantially less than for black youths.

## *DISCUSSION*

This analysis indicates that smoking blunts is a popular way to consume marijuana among youths nationwide. In 2000-03, about half of all marijuana users age 12-17 smoked blunts. Moreover, according to the 2002 NSDUH, more youths smoked blunts (5.1%) in the past-30-days than used cocaine in any form (1.2%), crack (0.2%), heroin (0.1%), ecstasy (0.4%) or methamphetamine (0.4%). Blunts were more common among blacks, older teens, males, and in metropolitan areas. These findings are consistent with qualitative evidence suggesting that smoking blunts has been centered in the inner-city Hip Hop culture. However, blunt smoking was also quite common among whites, females and in non-metropolitan areas indicating that by 2000 this practice had diffused widely. Moreover, the analysis of marijuana trend data indicated that the increase in marijuana use started at roughly the same time for

TABLE 4. Bivariate Variation in Past-30-Day Marijuana/Blunt Use Across Demographic Characteristics, NSDUH Respondents 2000-2003, Age 12-17

|  | Marijuana Use | Marijuana/Blunt Use | Blunt Use Given Marijuana/Blunt Use |
|---|---|---|---|
| *Age* |  |  |  |
| 12 years old | 0.7% | 1.0% | 48.4% |
| 13 years old | 1.9% | 2.7% | 52.3% |
| 14 years old | 5.2% | 6.2% | 50.5% |
| 15 years old | 9.8% | 11.3% | 50.3% |
| 16 years old | 13.3% | 15.2% | 56.4% |
| 17 years old | 16.4% | 18.5% | 58.4% |
| *Race/Ethnicity* |  |  |  |
| White | 8.5% | 9.6% | 50.7% |
| Black | 6.1% | 8.5% | 74.3% |
| Hispanic | 6.9% | 8.3% | 56.0% |
| Other | 6.5% | 6.9% | 52.2% |
| *Gender* |  |  |  |
| Male | 8.6% | 9.9% | 57.8% |
| Female | 7.0% | 8.2% | 50.9% |
| *MSA Size* |  |  |  |
| Over 1 million | 7.5% | 8.7% | 57.0% |
| Under 1 million | 8.4% | 9.9% | 56.2% |
| Not an MSA | 7.5% | 8.7% | 47.9% |
| *Interview Year* |  |  |  |
| 2000 | 7.2% | 8.4% | 54.9% |
| 2001 | 8.0% | 9.2% | 51.2% |
| 2002 | 8.2% | 9.3% | 58.1% |
| 2003 | 8.0% | 9.3% | 54.7% |

blacks and whites, and that the increase may have started earlier in areas that are not part of an MSA than in larger urban MSAs.

These results are consistent with the idea that the increase in youthful marijuana use during the 1990s was partially associated with the growing symbolic importance of blunts. However, it would appear that the popularity of marijuana use in other forms may have also been increasing and that the increase was not necessarily centered in the inner-city Hip Hop culture. To further investigate the role of blunts in fueling the increase in marijuana use, it would be very useful to ask young adults who reached their teens in the 1990s (currently age 18-35) if they ever smoked a blunt, their age at their first use, whether blunts were the first form in which they used marijuana, and the extent to which they consumed marijuana in other forms.

The NSDUH and other survey programs likely underestimated the increase in youthful marijuana use during the 1990s. Many youthful blunt smokers, especially blacks, appeared not to define blunt smoking as marijuana use when responding to the NSDUH; many respondents reported smoking blunts but not consuming marijuana. Adding in these respondents increased the prevalence of past-30-day marijuana use among 12-17 year olds by 16%. This addition also reduced the disparity in marijuana use between whites and blacks. These results suggest the NSDUH should be revised to explicitly indicate that marijuana can be smoked in a blunt or preferably to include parallel questions regarding use of blunts and of marijuana in other forms. Moreover, the data in Table 4 suggests that blunts use may be even more common among marijuana/blunts users who are age 18 and older. NSDUH (and other major surveys) should ask questions about blunt use among respondents 18 and older in the future.

Our findings also corroborated prior research that found youths tend not to define smoking blunts as cigar use (Yerger et al., 2001; Soldz et al., 2003). These findings provide further evidence that the increase in youthful cigar use during the 1990s was probably not due to youths reporting their smoking blunts as cigar use. It is possible, however, that youths' experiences with blunts and the popular culture references to these objects that look like cigars could have increased youths' familiarity and interest in cigars, as well as cigarettes and other conventional tobacco products. Further research into this topic is needed.

The current popularity of blunts has important implications for drug abuse prevention and treatment programs, particularly those that include a social behavior component. These programs typically seek to teach clients to deal with situations in which drug use may occur. This study suggests that to have credibility, especially among African American youths, these scenarios should address smoking blunts. More broadly, public health agencies need to identify the physical and mental health sequelae of blunt smoking and prepare to deal with them. The consequences of blunt smoking may differ from those associated with other forms of marijuana use. Moreover, there appears to be a large and growing cohort of blunt smokers that are accumulating years of this health risk behavior.

## NOTES

1. From 1990 to 1998, the NSDUH distinguished five categories of MSA size, but only three in other years. The "1/4 to 1 million" and "less than 1/4 million" categories were combined to match the "less than 1 million" category. The "rural area, not in an MSA" and "not in an MSA but not rural" rural categories were combined to match the "not in an MSA" category.

2. Given the large samples involved in these analyses, even small variations were identified as statistically significant, like the odds ratios of 0.9 associated with variation across interview years.

## REFERENCES

Alwin, D. F., & McCammon, R. J. (2003). Generations, cohorts and social change. In Mortimer, J. T. and Shanahan, M. J. (Eds.), *Handbook of the Life Course*. pp. 23-49. New York: Kluwer.

Biemer, P. P., Groves, R. M., Lyberg, L. E., Mathiowetz, N. A., & Sudman, S. (1991). Measurement Errors in Surveys. New York: Wiley.

Boehlert, E. (1994). Entertainment reporting spurs consumer spending. Billboard. February 5, 106, 36.

Community Epidemiology Work Group (1999). Identifying and Monitoring Emerging Drug Use Problems: A Retrospective Analysis of Drug Abuse Data/Information. Bethesda, MD: National Institute on Drug Abuse.

Del Boca, F., & Noll, J. E. (2000). Truth or consequences: The validity of self-report data in health services research on addictions. Addiction, 95 (Supplement 3), S347-S360.

Gfroerer, J., Eyerman, J., & Chromy, J. (Eds.) (2002). Redesigning an Ongoing National Household Survey: Methodological Issues. DHHS Publication No. SMA 03-3768. Rockville, MD: Substance Abuse and Mental Health Services Administration, Office of Applied Studies.

Gfroerer, J. C., Wu, L. T., & Penne, M. A. (2002) Initiation of Marijuana Use: Trends, Patterns, and Implications. DHHS Publication SMA 02-3711. Rockville, MD: Substance Abuse and Mental Health Services Administration, Office of Applied Studies.

Golub, A., & Johnson, B. D. (1997). Crack's decline: Some surprises across U.S. cities. Research in Brief, NCJ 165707. Washington, DC: National Institute of Justice.

Golub, A. L., & Johnson, B. D. (1999). Cohort changes in illegal drug use among arrestees in Manhattan: From the heroin injection generation to the blunts generation. Substance Use and Misuse, 34(13), pp. 1733-1763.

Golub, A., & Johnson, B. D. (2001). The rise of marijuana as the drug of choice among youthful adult arrestees. National Institute of Justice Research in Brief. NCJ 187490. Washington, DC: National Institute of Justice.

Golub, A., & Johnson, B. D. (2005). The new heroin users among Manhattan arrestees: Variations by race/ethnicity and mode of consumption. Journal of Psychoactive Drugs, 37(1), pp. 51-61.

Golub, A., Johnson, B. D., & Dunlap, E. (2005). Subcultural evolution and substance use. Addiction Research and Theory, 13(3), 217-229.

Golub, A., Johnson, B. D., Dunlap, E., & Sifaneck, S. (2004). Projecting and monitoring the life course of the marijuana/blunts generation. Journal of Drug Issues, 34(2), 361-388.

Golub, A., Johnson, B. D., Sifaneck, S., Chesluk, B., & Parker, H. (2001). Is the U.S. experiencing an incipient epidemic of hallucinogen use? Substance Use and Misuse, 36, 1699-1729.

Hosmer, D. W., & Lemeshow, S. (1989). Applied Logistic Regression. New York: Wiley.

Johnson, B. D., & Golub, A. L. (2002). Generational trends in heroin use and injection among arrestees in New York City. In Musto, D. (Ed.), One Hundred Years of Heroin. Westport, CT: Auburn House, pp. 91-128.

Johnson, B. D., Golub, A., & Dunlap, E. (2000). The rise and decline of hard drugs, drug markets and violence in New York City. In Blumstein, A. and Wallman, J., eds., The Crime Drop in America. New York: Cambridge, pp. 164-206.

Johnston, L. D., Bachman, J. G., & O'Malley, P. M. (2000). Monitoring the Future: A Continuing Study of American Youth (12th Grade Survey), 1999, Parts 1 through 7. Ann Arbor, MI: Institute for Social Research.

Johnston, L. D., O'Malley, P. M., & Bachman, J. G. (2003). Monitoring the Future National Survey Results on Drug Use, 1975-2002. Vol. 1. NIH Publication 03-5375. Bethesda, MD: National Institute on Drug Abuse.

Rogers, E. M. (1995). Diffusion of innovations, fourth edition. New York: Free Press.

Sifaneck, S. J., Kaplan, C. D., Dunlap, E., & Johnson, B. D. (2003). Blunts and blowtjes: Cannabis use practices in two cultural settings and their implications for secondary prevention. Journal of Free Inquiry in Creative Sociology, 31, 1-11.

Soldz, S., Huyser, D. J., & Dorsey, E. (2003). The cigar as a drug delivery device: Youth use of blunts. Addiction, 98, 1379-1386.

Substance Abuse and Mental Health Services Administration [SAMHSA]. (1996). The Development and Implementation of a New Data Collection Instrument for the 1994 National Household Survey on Drug Abuse. Rockville, MD: Department of Health and Human Services. DHHS Publication No. (SMA) 96-3084. Available at www.samhsa.gov.

Substance Abuse and Mental Health Services Administration. (2000). National House-hold Survey on Drug Abuse, 1998, Codebook. Rockville, MD: Office of Applied Studies, Substance Abuse and Mental Health Services Administration.

Substance Abuse and Mental Health Services Administration. (2001). Summary of Findings from the 2000 National Household Survey on Drug Abuse: Vol. 1. Summary of National Findings (NHSDA Series H-13). DHHS Publication SMA 01-3549. Rockville, MD: Office of Applied Studies, Substance Abuse and Mental Health Services Administration.

Substance Abuse and Mental Health Services Administration. (2002a). National Household Survey on Drug Abuse, 1999, Codebook. Rockville, MD: Office of Applied Studies, Substance Abuse and Mental Health Services Administration.

Substance Abuse and Mental Health Services Administration (2002b). Results from the 2001 National Household Survey on Drug Abuse: Vol. 1. Summary of National Findings (NHSDA Series H-17). NIH Publication SMA 02-3758. Rockville, MD: Substance Abuse and Mental Health Services Administration, Office of Applied Studies.

Substance Abuse and Mental Health Services Administration. (2002c). National Household Survey on Drug Abuse, 2000, Codebook. Rockville, MD: Office of Applied Studies, Substance Abuse and Mental Health Services Administration.

Substance Abuse and Mental Health Services Administration. (2003a). The National Survey on Drug Use and Health. NHSDA Report. February 7. Rockville, MD: Substance Abuse and Mental Health Services Administration, Office of Applied Studies.

Substance Abuse and Mental Health Services Administration. (2003b). National Household Survey on Drug Abuse, 2001, Codebook. Rockville, MD: Office of Applied Studies, Substance Abuse and Mental Health Services Administration.

Substance Abuse and Mental Health Services Administration (2003c). Results from the 2002 National Household Survey on Drug Abuse: National Findings (NHSDA Series H-22). NIH Publication SMA 03-3836. Rockville, MD.

Substance Abuse and Mental Health Services Administration. (2004a). National Household Survey on Drug Abuse, 2002, Codebook. Rockville, MD: Office of Applied Studies, Substance Abuse and Mental Health Services Administration.

Substance Abuse and Mental Health Services Administration. (2004b). National Household Survey on Drug Abuse, 2003, Codebook. Rockville, MD: Office of Applied Studies, Substance Abuse and Mental Health Services Administration.

Yerger, V., Pearson, C., & Malone, R. E. (2001). When is a cigar not a cigar? African American youths' understanding of "cigar" use. American Journal of Public Health, 91, 316-317.

# Cigars-for-Blunts:
# Choice of Tobacco Products by Blunt Smokers

Stephen J. Sifaneck, PhD
Bruce D. Johnson, PhD
Eloise Dunlap, PhD

**SUMMARY.** An important part of blunt (marijuana in a cigar shell) smoking is the ritual of the preparation process and the selection of tobacco product for the blunt. This article explores reasons for selection from the different tobacco products available in the legal commercial market. Based upon three years of ethnographic research with 92 focal subjects, the analysis focuses upon the practical, subcultural, and symbolic reasons that blunt smokers give for choosing tobacco products (cigars for blunts–CFBs) employed in the blunt preparation process. The blunt ritual also functions within the marijuana subculture to differentiate blunt smokers from joints/pipes smokers.

---

Stephen J. Sifaneck, Bruce D. Johnson, and Eloise Dunlap are affiliated with National Development and Research Institutes, Inc., New York, NY.

The authors acknowledge the many contributions of Flutura Bardhi, Anthony Nguyen, Doris Randolph, and Ricardo Bracho.

This research was funded by the National Institute on Drug Abuse (NIDA–5R01 DA 013690-04) to study blunts/marijuana use patterns, social, economic, and physical contexts where consumption of marijuana occurs, and the marijuana market. Additional support is provided by other projects (R01 DA09056-10, T32 DA07233-21).

The ideas or points of view in this paper do not represent the official position of the U.S. Government, National Institute on Drug Abuse, or National Development and Research Institutes Inc.

[Haworth co-indexing entry note]: "Cigars-for-Blunts: Choice of Tobacco Products by Blunt Smokers." Sifaneck, Stephen J., Bruce D. Johnson, and Eloise Dunlap. Co-published simultaneously in *Journal of Ethnicity in Substance Abuse* (The Haworth Press, Inc.) Vol. 4, No. 3/4, 2005, pp. 23-42; and: *The Cultural/Subcultural Contexts of Marijuana Use at the Turn of the Twenty-First Century* (ed: Andrew Golub) The Haworth Press, Inc., 2005, pp. 23-42. Single or multiple copies of this article are available for a fee from The Haworth Document Delivery Service [1-800-HAWORTH, 9:00 a.m. - 5:00 p.m. (EST). E-mail address: docdelivery@haworthpress. com].

This analysis explores the reasons users give for selecting among the most popular inexpensive cigar brands (Dutch Masters, Phillies Blunts, and Backwoods) all owned and marketed by a single cigar conglomerate. "Blunt chasing"–the smoking of a cigarillo or cigar following a blunt–is an emergent phenomenon that further expands the market for tobacco products among blunt smokers. Recently, many different flavors have been added to these tobacco products in order to attract young and minority blunt consumers. *[Article copies available for a fee from The Haworth Document Delivery Service: 1-800-HAWORTH. E-mail address: <docdelivery@haworthpress.com> Website: <http://www.HaworthPress.com>* © 2005 by The Haworth Press, Inc. All rights reserved.]*

**KEYWORDS.** Blunts, cigars, marijuana, tobacco, minority, youth, subculture

## INTRODUCTION

Blunts have become a very common mode of consumption among marijuana users. An important part of blunt smoking is the ritual of the preparation process. One integral part of the preparation process is the selection of the tobacco product to make the blunt. This article will explore users reasons for selection from the different tobacco products available in the legal commercial market. A blunt is made by wrapping marijuana in the shell of a low cost cigar or sheet of tobacco, and is smoked like a marijuana joint. Blunts have become a common way in which marijuana is consumed by young persons in New York City and other urban and non-urban parts of the United States (Golub, Johnson, Dunlap, 2005). While marketing of marijuana remains illegal, marketing cigars (for adults) remains legal. The inexpensive cigars commonly used to make blunts (Phillies Blunts, White Owls, Dutch Masters, Backwoods) are generally not smoked by cigar aficionados nor sold at upscale cigar stores; rather, these products can be observed being sold alongside cigarettes and other tobacco products at delis, bodegas, supermarkets, package stores, newsstands, and gas stations.

Altadis U.S.A. markets over 100 brands of cigars and 20 brands of low cost cigarillos. Altadis U.S.A. sponsors a website with a complete listing of its products and a history of the company (www.altadisusa.com). Further, Altadis markets the most common cigar products used by blunt smokers: Phillies Blunts, Dutch Masters, and Backwoods. They have also introduced flavored versions of their traditional cigar products. About five years ago, smaller tobacco companies introduced an entirely new tobacco product, labeled as *blunt wraps*, which are solely intended and labeled for purchase by blunt smokers. Despite disclaimers such as "for smoking tobacco only," blunt wraps cannot be smoked alone; they serve as a delivery system for another smoked product. Blunts smokers interviewed for this research clearly understood that marijuana is smoked in a blunt wrap. These smaller more independent tobacco companies that sell blunt wraps have also included flavors in their product line.

This paper addresses some specific questions concerning the tobacco products that youths choose when smoking blunts. What are some of the practical and symbolic reasons for their choice of a cigar-for-blunts (henceforth CFB)? What impact has the tobacco flavoring trend had on these choices, especially regarding young novice and minority blunt smokers? This article explores these practical reasons exploring issues involved in sharing, preparation, concealment of use, and flavor enhancement. This paper will also explore the many symbolic connections between CFBs and blunt smoking, to the social worlds of street culture (Hip Hop), alcohol, and nightlife.

At a theoretical level, blunt smoking and associated rituals provide important insights about the continuing evolution and changes within drug subcultures (Johnson, 1980; Golub, Johnson, & Dunlap, 2005). The ways that marijuana rituals help delineate especially common use patterns constitute important "boundaries" or "differentiation" within the international community of marijuana users. In the United States, a widely recognized form of marijuana consumption has involved rolling marijuana in cigarette paper and smoking it as a "joint." Consumption via a variety of pipes (e.g., glass, bongs, bubblers) is also common among joint users. This American "joint/pipe" subculture is relatively unique in excluding tobacco products from marijuana use practices. In most of Europe, the term "joint" means using cigarette paper to roll a mixture of marijuana with loose-leaf tobacco; this is called a "blowtje" in the Netherlands (Sifaneck & Kaplan, 1995; Sifaneck et al., 2003). Among West Indians, spliffs (marijuana rolled in a true tobacco leaf) are the common consumption unit (Hamid, 2000). While outsiders (nonusers and policy makers) may consider such use rituals as relatively unimportant or irrelevant, the distinctive rituals for consuming marijuana constitute important symbolic and practical considerations among committed users. Indeed, within each of these different traditions, considerable discussion and opinions occurs among committed marijuana users about the relative merits of using different commercial products (e.g., brand of cigarette paper, types of tobacco leaf, loose leaf tobacco) as part of the smoking rituals.

Among the blunt users analyzed below, participation in rituals of choosing CFBs, their skill at rolling blunts, and sharing consumption of blunts constitutes (in many symbolic ways) the very definition of their group–as blunt users–and many consider themselves to be quite distinct from "joint/pipe users." Their choice of cigars-for-blunts matters a great deal to blunt users, although their brand preferences are influenced by many other symbolic factors (naming of cigars, flavoring, music, and lifestyle considerations, etc.) described below. The focus of this article is upon respondents' explanation about the choice of specific tobacco products with which to roll blunts.

## THE BLUNT USE PHENOMENON

"Blunts" explicitly emerged as a phenomenon in New York City during the mid 1980s, where small groups (3-5) of youth would pool their limited resources to purchase generally a "dime" ($10) or "nickel" ($5) bag of marijuana. During the late 1980s, New York City's inner-city markets offered relatively small amounts: a nickel consisting of approximately 0.75 gram, and a dime averaging slightly more than 1.5 grams. When rolling a traditional marijuana joint, 1 gram might be used to construct 2-3 slim joints wrapped in cigarette paper. Joints of this size were usually consumed by one or two persons (Sifaneck et al., 2003).

The blunt smoking phenomenon emerged from a number of social forces (Johnson et al., 1990; Johnson, Golub, & Dunlap, 2000; Sifaneck et al., 2003). When making a blunt, the user purchases an inexpensive, low-quality cigar. "Phillies Blunts" from which the *blunt* label is derived, is one popular commercial brand, but other cheap cigars (i.e., White Owls, Dutch Masters, and Backwoods) are also widely used by blunt smokers. The exterior shell of these low cost cigars is a tobacco/glue/paper composite that can be cleanly cut with a sharp edge. Unlike higher priced cigars, these shells are not made of broad leaf tobacco, which crumbles when cut.

The ritual of the blunt rolling process has many variations and is relatively simple, but does require a certain amount of acquired skill and practice. The low-cost cigar is moistened with saliva and then split length-wise down the center with either a fingernail or knife blade; the tobacco inside is emptied out. The shell is reduced or shortened to about two-thirds of the original cigar's length. The shell is then moistened thoroughly with saliva. This is done for two reasons: (1) to release the adhesive qualities of the glue in the shell, and (2) to make the shell more pliable and easy to roll. The cigar shell is then re-filled with marijuana and rolled up. The completed blunt looks like a large cigarette or a half-size cigar. Generally, a whole dime ($10 worth) of marijuana is used in the construction, and the blunt is often shared by a group of three or more users. Since blunts have come into fashion, however, individual blunt smoking among wealthier users is not uncommon. The original blunt smokers of the mid 1980s, predominantly African-Caribbean, African-American, and Latino youth residing in the inner-city neighborhoods of New York, perceived their new method of (blunt) preparation as an economical way to consume marijuana. It has also become a valuable ritual involving a group market transaction and preparation process (Dunlap et al., this volume).

The marijuana leaf symbol has become a generalized *icon* representing the marijuana subculture. Persons who wear the marijuana leaf symbol on their clothing effectively announce their willingness to use it and probable opposition to marijuana prohibition. In a similar fashion, the shape of the blunt or cigar, and the words *blunts*, *Phillies*, and *Dutches* have become icons that symbolize the blunts subculture in several ways; the very name "blunts" comes from a brand-named cigar, Phillies Blunts. The word "Phillie" (often misspelled as Philly) is equivalent to a cigar shell containing marijuana. A cigar in many music videos and other forms of advertising is understood by blunt subculture members as a visual reference–an icon–for blunt smoking itself.

Indeed, the image and use of blunts became an integral element in the "Hip-Hop" youth subculture that has emerged in most American cities. Other elements of this subculture include rap music, dance styles, a continuously evolving argot (including unique terms for marijuana), graffiti art, and styles of dress that include baggy pants, sport team jackets and caps, oversized jewelry, and a changing array of accessories. Hats and shirts with the "Phillies Blunts" logo, and other references to blunts and marijuana smoking are common icons displayed prominently on "street gear" or the apparel of Hip-Hop. The argot of the Hip-Hop subculture includes many novel and innovative terms for marijuana (i.e., chronic, ism, boom, live, lah, dro). Blunt smokers rarely use terms such as pot, reefer, Mary Jane, grass–and consider these terms obsolete. The new argot serves the function of concealing conversations about marijuana from persons who are not members of the blunts subculture and integrating those so involved (Johnson et al., 2005).

Rap songs offer instructions about how to roll blunts and smoke them. Phallic shaped blunts are also an expression of "phatness." "Phat" or "fat" is an important symbolic concept for the Hip-Hop subculture and analogous to excellent. Blunts are one expression of "phat," as are "forties" (40-ounce bottles of beer or malt-liquor), and oversized baggy pants and sweatshirts. Phat is essentially a subcultural expression of "living large"; what the media has termed "ghetto fabulous." Since a blunt is essentially a large or phat "joint," it constitutes a central symbolic expression of this phatness. Blunts are a particular mode of consumption, and also an important expression of how new marijuana users see themselves as different from older marijuana using subcultures. In previous marijuana subcultures (e.g., Hippie, Rastafarianism) more common modes of consumption were joints and spliffs, and to a lesser extent bongs and pipes. Gemi, a 19-year-old Japanese-American male blunt smoker who identifies with the Hip Hop subculture, explains the practical and subcultural reasons he prefers blunts over other ways of smoking marijuana:

> It's tradition, man. [laughs] It's like you have to . . . you have the cigar; you get the cigar and then you break it up. And then, you know, I pride myself . . . a good roller. I make a nice clean L [blunt], that smokes well. And, um, so for tradition's sake, I guess. And you know, pipes and bongs are kinda like, they're not as like, um, I don't know, mobile. And, um, I don't really hang with people who smoke a lot of pipes. I haven't been out to the west coast in a while, and I don't hang out with too many white people, so. You know. Blunts is the order of the day.

In this quote, Gemi discusses the symbolic and practical reasons blunt smoking is important to him. On the practical side he sees blunts as a portable and "mobile" way to consume marijuana. On the symbolic level he sees his blunt smoking as identifying with East Coast Hip Hop and street culture. In the discussion to follow, other practical and symbolic considerations impact upon user decisions in choosing a CFB for blunt smoking.

## *METHODS*

Based on observations and interviews during a three-year ethnographic study, entitled Marijuana/Blunts: Use, Markets, and Subcultures, staff has documented how blunt use is widely prevalent in most New York City neighborhoods, as is the "cigars-for-blunts" phenomenon. Ethnographic staff recruited subjects between the ages of 14 and 35 who would represent the diverse experiences of marijuana/blunt users based on age, race/ethnicity, gender and class/neighborhood. Project management hired ethnographers who are demographically diverse in terms of age, race (black, white, Latino, and Asian), gender and sexual orientation. This diversity aided in the access to different groups of marijuana/blunt users, and in the initial rapport project ethnographers could develop with potential subjects. Ethnographers attempted to diversify the respondent pool by seeking individuals who identified with various subcultures, were raised and "hung out" in different locations, and were from diverse ethnic backgrounds.

Respondents in the sample included several high school-aged subjects, and they differed in their backgrounds and experiences. They attended both public and private high schools located in midtown, downtown, and even so far as Riverdale in the Bronx. Several who had dropped out of high school were also located and recruited. These youthful respondents associated themselves with various subcultural groups, such as graffiti artists, skateboarders, automobile enthusiasts, and hippies. Some students had recently completed their college application process, while others were in the midst of taking their PSATs and SATs and beginning to prepare their own college selection process. Other students struggled with the prospect of finishing school and earning their high school diploma. Recruiting persons under the age of 18 years required project staff to obtain parental consent. The parental consent form presented the study as investigating "smoking behaviors" among youth. Describing the study as such was not misleading, and allowed minors to avoid implicitly disclosing their marijuana use to their parents or guardians.

College students in the sample represented a range of respondents from public and private universities located in the city. Subjects included writers, actors, filmmakers, fine artists, communications majors, computer programmers, sculptors, musicians, fashion designers, party promoters, and community activists. While many lived in student housing dispersed across downtown Manhattan, a number of college students lived in privately rented apartments in neighborhoods in Manhattan, Brooklyn and Queens. The sample also included a number of young adults who were finished with their college studies, and often were part of the city's workforce. These occupations included writers, fashion designers, artists, bar and restaurant workers, and office staff workers.

The smoking behaviors of subjects also covered a broad range of smoking patterns, activities, practices, and rituals. Over the course of three years of observation, respondents had variable use patterns that shifted across time. Methods of smoking and preferences differed, as well: while many subjects had smoked marijuana in a variety of modes including blunts, bongs, joints, bubblers (a hybrid of a glass pipe and a bong), pipes made from hollowed apples, pipes made from soda cans, one hitters (hollowed tubes disguised as cigarettes), vaporizers (devices that heat marijuana until it vaporizes), and even eaten marijuana in brownies, cookies, or popcorn, several subjects expressed strict preferences in terms of how they smoked or consumed marijuana. Some swore by blunts, while others disdained them in favor of pipes or joints.

Field staff initially interviewed 120 subjects of different races, ages, and genders. From this larger sample 92 respondents were chosen as focal subjects for an in-depth baseline interview and follow-up interviews that took place every 6 months. The focal subject sample is 43% female, 32% white, 24% African-American, 19% Latino, and 14% Asian. A quarter exclusively used blunts; a tenth report exclusively using marijuana but not as blunts. Two-thirds reported using both blunts and joints/pipes. Reasons given for these preferences were varied and included reasons concerning taste, the inclusion of tobacco as in the case of blunts, and the importance of social rituals.

The in-depth baseline interview schedule employed during the course of the data collection phase of the study encompassed a number of substantive areas of inquiry. Its main intent was to measure the current and past use of marijuana/blunts, alcohol, tobacco, as well as to ascertain subcultural conduct norms and contexts of marijuana/blunt use. The other main focus of the baseline interview schedule involved extended life-histories from our respondents. Issues concerning life experiences growing up, including family life, neighborhood environments, and family members' use of drugs and alcohol were all included. We also explored present day issues regarding lifestyle, subcultural influences, sexual behaviors, and potential criminal and violent behaviors. Interviews were audio taped, professionally transcribed, and generally lasted between 60 and 90 minutes. Follow-up interviews focused on changes in the subject's use of marijuana, tobacco, alcohol and other drugs, as well as other changes that occurred with the subject over the last six months.

The development of the ethnographic interview guides did not begin before preliminary ethnographic fieldwork. Staff of the project performed naturalistic observations of marijuana/blunt users in various contexts, making note of the social rituals and material products that were part of the smoking process. Informal in the field interviews were performed with users, dealers, and non-marijuana-using peers. From these insights collected in the field, questions for the depth interview instrument were developed with an "ethnographic sensitivity." This sensitivity included: (1) constructing questions as they would be delivered in a normal conversation, avoiding terms that would sound judgmental or clinical; (2) using words that were "youth-friendly" but also understood by older users; and (3) developing questions that suggested that we were familiar with subject matter and its subcultural nuances. Making sure questions were ethnographically sensitive for a heterogeneous sample of marijuana users was quite a challenge, since this sensitivity included many layers of subcultural understanding. Subcultural meanings, language, and symbolisms were routinely shared at bi-monthly staff meetings. Sharing this information in a routine and systematic way served to keep staff ethnographers "in the know" about the various social networks other staff ethnographers were exploring.

An important analytical construction was included in the interview schedules: the distinction between marijuana use in a joint, pipe, or bong and marijuana use that involved a blunt. This distinction between "marijuana" smoked in other ways (mainly "joints") and marijuana smoked as "blunts" was useful on a number of levels. A central issue whether use patterns, social rituals, and signs of dependency would differ between our respondents who smoked marijuana outside of the blunt format and users who smoked marijuana in the form of blunts. It is interesting that this distinction has been recognized by survey analysts who contend that youthful respondents may often not "define blunt smoking as marijuana use" (Golub, Johnson, & Dunlap, 2005, this volume; Soldz, Huyser, & Dorsey, 2003).

Ethnographic research has its limitations. It is more suited for developing hypotheses, than substantiating them. Even though staff systematically attempted to include various types of marijuana/blunt users in our sample, it is likely that every type of user is not adequately represented. Since marijuana is a drug that intersects with so many different social groups and lifestyles recruiting an ethnographic sample inclusive of every type of user would be a difficult task. The ethnographic data that is presented was collected from a diverse group of young marijuana and blunt users in New York City.

Subjects were asked the question: "What type of cigars do you purchase to make your blunts with?" They were then probed about different CFBs and other tobacco products such as blunt wraps and fronto leaf. Some focal subjects were later probed about the reasons for their CFB choice. In this article we will first provide a brief explanation of the blunt use phenomenon. Discussion of the tobacco products utilized by blunt smokers will follow, with an emphasis on the new flavored products available on the market. Finally, we will address the implications of these tobacco products regarding youth and minorities.

## TOBACCO PRODUCTS FOR BLUNT SMOKING

### Cigars-For-Blunts (CFBs)

When blunts emerged as a phenomenon in New York City and elsewhere, the tobacco products used in the construction of blunts were relatively limited. Most young inner-city blunt users opted to use the cigar from which the "blunt" label is derived: the Phillies Blunt. These inexpensive cigars were sold at delis, newsstands, and bodegas throughout the city. The retail cost of $0.50 made it affordable for most blunt users. As the blunt rolling practice developed and matured, and as blunt smoking gained popularity, the range of inexpensive cigars used by blunt smokers–the Cigars-For-Blunts (CFB) market–expanded. White Owl and Optimo cigars were two brands that competed with the Phillies Blunt. In the late 1980s these two brands were also sold at neighborhood delis and bodegas for $0.50, the same price as the Phillies Blunt. "Dutch Masters" are the latest cigars which have emerged as a popular choice among blunt smokers and they presently sell for $1.00-$1.25 each in most New York City neighborhoods. The popularity of Dutch Masters cigars used to make blunts was widely reported. Preliminary analysis of limited survey data[1] with blunt smokers in New York found that three quarters reported using Dutch Masters, over half reported using Phillies Blunts, about a sixth reported White Owl and Backwoods, with less than 5% reported use of Optimos. A constantly evolving urban street mythology explains effects of the highs, the burning duration, and reasons for choosing among the different brands. Marley,[2] a 28-year-old Irish-American with dreadlocks, a long-time blunt smoker and party promoter, explains her choice of cigar for rolling blunts:

Dutch Masters. I've rolled them all. Sometimes I go into a little phase where I like Garcia Vega. And a lot of my dreads (Rastafarians), they roll Backwoods. It's just like a Jamaican thing. But pretty much Dutch Masters. Phillies was the first that I rolled, and I was true to them for a long time. But there's something about the Dutch Master, the extra step of having to do the leaf and everything that kind of makes it the thing to roll right now. With a Dutch Master rolling is more of a specialty; because you got to peel the outer layer first, then empty it and then repack it and then re-roll it. And it looks like an original cigar that you're smoking.

It is clear that Marley has carefully considered her brand options for choosing a cigar to make blunts. The fact that Marley can produce a blunt from a Dutch Masters that looks much like the original cigar seems to be of paramount importance. This quality provides a number of functions. First if the blunt produced looks like a cigar it makes it easier to consume in an inconspicuous manner. Second, a blunt that resembles the original cigar is evidence of Marley's acquired and acute blunt rolling skills. This skill gives her status within the blunt smoking subculture. Three of the four cigar brands she mentions (Dutch Masters, Phillies, and Backwoods) are marketed by Altadis U.S.A. She also mentions the symbolic importance of Backwoods with Rastafarians, which will be explored later in the paper.

Mary Jane, a 25-year-old African-American female blunt smoker from Harlem, explains the constantly changing selection involved in the cigars for blunts market, comparing the choice of a CFB, to a consumer choice of music genres:

It's like with weed . . . smoking's a fad, too, just like Hip Hop. And it's like during certain times, it's popular to smoke certain things. And if like people is only smoking the Phillies at that time, it's wack for you to smoke in a White Owl. Like, what you doing smoking in a White Owl? That's old school. Like now Dutches (Dutch Masters) is in. And if you see a person smoking in a Philly, you'll think they're an old head. Like they back, you been smoking since the 80s, smoking in a Philly. You know, like that's ancient.

Mary Jane invokes the role of peer influence when selecting a CFB, which is also a factor when youth choose a brand of cigarette to smoke. Youth often smoke the same brands their friends smoke. Mary Jane also speaks to the generational subcultural status involved in a choice of a

CFB. She suggests younger users are more likely to choose a CFB that is popular at the moment (in this case Dutch Masters), as one might choose a recording artist to listen to. Selection of a White Owl or a Phillies Blunt would suggest the blunt smoker was of an older generation of blunt users, and is not as in touch with current trends in CFB choices. The reasons she mentions for choosing a CFB have nothing to do with any of the practical considerations of blunt smoking, and are focused around the symbolic status represented by purchasing and smoking the more expensive CFB, which Dutch Masters currently represents.

Backwoods cigars are a tobacco product that emerged on the market in the mid-1990s and have competed formidably among blunt smokers as an alternative to other inexpensive cigars such as Phillies Blunts, White Owls, and Dutch Masters. Backwoods, unlike other low-cost cigars, claim to be one hundred percent tobacco; the shell is not a paper/tobacco/glue composite. This quality makes a blunt rolled with a Backwoods shell closer to the experience of smoking a spliff (marijuana rolled inside "fronto leaf"–a true tobacco leaf). Blunt smokers who prefer Backwoods for making blunts perceive themselves as tobacco "purists" in that the cigar they are using is not a processed one. Backwoods are quite popular among adherents of the Rastafarian subculture who avoid "processed" products and perceive Backwoods as "more natural" (Hamid, 2002). Loco Bravo, a white 25-year-old regular blunt and joint smoker, believes this "natural" product compromises his health less: "It doesn't feel quite as dirty in my lungs. Not as dirty as other cigars." The health concerns involved in Loco Bravos choice are similar to the health-related sentiments expressed by those identifying with the Rastafarian subculture. Roy Earl, a 28-year-old Irish/Columbian blunt smoker, a skateboarder who works for an independent record label and is originally from the North West coast, expresses more practical reasons for why he chooses Backwoods:

> I smoke Backwoods 'cause I like the way it feels. The paper is really thin, and feels more natural, not like all the thick paper that you get when you roll a Dutch or a Philly, where it's all cumbersome to roll, although, don't get me wrong, I can still roll 'em. I like the way it burns too, and the way it pulls: it's a cleaner and crisper feel and I don't feel like I am wrecking my lungs as much when I smoke, because those chemicals you find in the other cigars just aren't there. I know they (Backwoods) came out with all those new flavors, but I think I am gonna stick with the Sweet and Aromatic kind, although I am a little intrigued by how a Backwoods Strawberry would taste.

Similar to Loco Bravo, whose reasons for choosing Backwoods seemed entirely health-related, Roy Earl also coincides with these sentiments, attributing the "chemicals" in other brands as potentially harmful to health, but also expresses practical reasons for selecting Backwoods as a CFB. He suggests they are easier to roll than the other CFB brands, and he believes the blunts made from a Backwoods "burn" and "pull" better than their competitors, thus providing a more efficient delivery system for the smoked marijuana.

Dutch Masters was the most popular brand reported by our respondents. Users often had very specific reasons why they paid the extra 25-50 cents for a Dutch Masters. One reason for its popularity was that the sheet of tobacco was longer in length and easier to roll with. T-Bone, an 18 year-old Puerto Rican blunt smoker, explained, "Dutch is the best thing to roll with because if you mess up the first time you roll they have enough leaf to cover if you got a hole in your blunt." Bird, a 29-year-old blunt smoker of mixed race, who works in street culture marketing, explains his reasons for smoking Dutch Masters at the present time in his marijuana use career:

> Dutch Masters. Um, through my phases in life, the first few years was only Phillies. Um, thousands of them. And then, um, I got into Dutch Masters, a couple thousand of those. And then I got into Garcia Vegas. And then Garcia Vegas changed how they wrap the cigars, so I went back to Dutch Masters, Grenadines, Optimo Grenadines. But mostly Dutch Master.

Bird is also an example how blunt users choice in CFBs changes over the course of ones blunt smoking career, and may be affected by practical considerations such as packaging. The importance of the freshness of tobacco products used to make blunts, in terms of taste and "rolling utility" or playability, was a recurring theme in the interviews. The new way that Garcia Vegas were packaged did not meet the freshness standards of Bird, and this ultimately affected his CFB choice.

### Flavored Cigars for Blunt Smoking

Tobacco control experts have been cognizant of new flavor added cigarettes, but little attention has been placed on flavored tobacco products used for making *blunts*. Recent analyses have focused on how tobacco companies are appealing to youthful and minority customers by adding "sweet" and "spicy" flavors to their cigarettes. In 2002, RJ

Reynolds introduced a line of Camel brand cigarettes called "Exotic Flavors" which included flavors "Berry Bayou Blast," "Crema Mint," "Koula Kolada," and "Twista Lime." In 2004, Brown and Williamson released the Kool Smooth Fusion line of cigarettes including flavors like "Mintrigue," "Midnight Berry," and "Mocha Taboo." These new flavored cigarettes have been designed to directly appeal to young and novice cigarette users, to help regain consumers they may have lost (Connolly, 2004).

Recently, cigars such as Phillies Blunt and Dutch Masters have become available in different flavors. Both of these cigar brands, popular for making blunts, represent a fair share of the Cigars for Blunts market. Blunt smokers perceive these as competing brands, and are probably unaware they are marketed by the same cigar company (Altadis, U.S.A.). Based on observations at retail stores that sell cigars in New York City, a continuously expanding selection of new flavors has occurred over the past three years. Phillies Blunt was first available in "Strawberry Daiquiri" flavor, a sweetened alcoholic/rum taste that seems to be a direct appeal to young women and Latino blunt smokers. This flavor is very similar to the "Koula Kolada" in the Camel cigarette line of "Exotic Flavors" in the sense it is flavored with a sweet fruit- and rum-like taste. Both Daiquiris and (Pina) (K)Coladas are sweet rum-based beverages seemingly favored by women and young novice drinkers. Moreover, marijuana users are likely to use alcohol, often at the same time. These new alcoholic flavored tobacco products for smoking blunts are targeted strategically at both young alcohol and marijuana consumers who are beginning to establish preferences for specific brands and flavors of cigars for blunts.

Altadis U.S.A. now manufactures Phillies Blunt cigars in a dozen flavors: Banana, Berry, Chocolate, Cinnamon, Coconut, Cognac, Green de menthe, Honey, Peach, Sour Apple, Strawberry, and Vanilla. The Phillies Blunt brand has also introduced "Phillies Barrel O'Blunts Cigars" in several flavors which are cans of fifty cigars. Dutch Masters are available in chocolate, vanilla and honey flavors, known respectively on the street as "chocolate Dutch," "vanilla Dutch," and "honey Dutch." Both Phillies Blunt and Dutch Masters first offered their products in only one flavored variety. The fact that both CFBs are now offered in multiple flavors indicates that the marketing on the initial flavor was successful. Backwoods is also now available in Regular, Sweet Aromatic, Black N Sweet, Wild Rum, and the new Honey and Honey Berry.

Snake, a white 17-year-old blunt smoker, is a fan of flavored cigars:

> Phillies come in all flavors. I've had vanilla, strawberry, sour apple, honey, chocolate. And Dutch Masters come different, too. There's like cognac flavored Dutches, vanilla, regular Dutch Master, and corona.

Flavored cigars and blunt wraps are favored by some blunt smokers, and avoided by others. The flavoring makes the taste of the blunt sweeter, masking the bitter taste of the tobacco and/or the marijuana. These flavored cigars for blunts appear to be targeting the young, female, and minority market niches. The flavoring also serves to mask the smell of the marijuana when the blunt is smoked. Bright Eyes, a 17 year-old African-American female from Harlem, explains why she chooses a flavored cigar:

> Vanilla Dutch. That's my favorite. It's not too heavy when you burn it, it make it smell like you smoking a cigarette . . . when somebody passes you they can't tell.

Bright Eyes implies the "cover-up" effect that the flavoring provides the burning blunt. When un-flavored blunts are smoked, the tobacco may also help mask the smell of the burning marijuana. When the flavor is added the marijuana smell is masked even more. This is a very important function that blunt smoking provides as opposed to other ways of smoking marijuana. Since the public use of marijuana has been considered a Quality of Life Crime (Golub et al., 2003), where users caught often spend the night in a holding cell, young marijuana smokers who use outdoors have to be extra careful that their use is not detected. Blunts have assisted in providing smoke that masks the relatively pungent smell of marijuana, thus, misleading passersby and police about what is really being smoked. Blunt users report their perceptions that flavored CFBs and blunt wraps help them conceal their consumption and possession of an illicit drug, especially in public locations.

### Blunt Wraps

"Blunt Wraps" are equal to the outer shell of a low-cost cigar, and have no possible intended purpose except to construct a blunt. This shell is what the blunt smoker is seeking to use when s/he dismantles and discards the filler of the low-cost cigars described previously. In a sense blunt wraps are useful to novice blunt smokers, since half of the blunt construction process is eliminated. Presently there are several tobacco companies that market blunts wraps. These tobacco products are not produced by the major tobacco companies, nor by the cigar giant Altadis, but by at least 9 smaller, more independent tobacco companies. The manufacturers of blunt wraps include: 420 Blunts, Amico Flavored Wraps, Blunt EZ, Blunt Wrap Brand, Flavored Blunt Cones, Golden Wraps, Loose Blunts, Royal Blunts, and True Blunts.

Blunt wraps are available in a wide range of conventional flavors such as chocolate, strawberry, vanilla, honey, and cognac, and other flavors that are more image-oriented–which directly appeal to the tastes of adolescents, young women, and minority youth. Some of the available flavors such as "Cotton Candy" and "Bubble Gum" seem to be directly marketed toward very young novice users. Other flavors such as "Gin and Juice," "Cognac" and "Crystal" are inspired by alcoholic beverages popular within the Hip Hop subculture. This type of subcultural target marketing is similar to the Kool Smooth Fusions cigarettes introduced in 2004, with flavors celebrating Hip-Hop and nightlife lifestyle: "Mintrigue," "Midnight Berry," and "Mocha Taboo."

The most popular reason reported for making a blunt with a blunt wrap was practical: the convenience and ease of not having to disassemble the cigar. Mori, a white 25-year-old female blunt smoker, and recent college graduate, articulates the convenience of blunt wraps:

> I also buy the packages, these things called Royal Blunts (a brand of blunt wrap). There's a couple of brands, and they come with just the paper, just the wrap, kind of like fronto leaf. It's processed tobacco, but it's not a cigar, so you don't have to get rid of the inside. It's just what you need. It's just a wrap.

Even though some respondents reported using blunt wraps, far more users reported using the shell of an inexpensive cigar to construct their blunts. Those who reported that they avoid the use of blunt wraps did so for number of reasons. Many users expressed the fact that dismantling the cigar was an important part of the blunt-making ritual, an important symbolic activity that separates the blunt subculture from the joints/pipes subculture. Many users saw the construction of the blunt as important as the actual smoking of the blunt; disassembling of the cigar was an integral part of the blunt construction process. Some users complained that blunt wraps did not sell as quickly as the blunt-making cigars, and were often too dry and stale to make a proper blunt. Recently blunt wraps have become available in more air-tight packaging to insure their freshness. Other users also reported that the tobacco sheets of the blunt wraps are too thick, and therefore produce a blunt that tastes too harsh. Some respondents reported that only novices without proper blunt rolling skills resort to using blunt wraps.

Unlike the inexpensive cigars used to make blunts, blunt wraps are more likely to be sold in head shops, or stores that sell marijuana paraphernalia (still legal and tolerated in New York City), or in tobacco shops that sell a selection of cigars. Thus, youth's access to blunt wraps may be far more restricted than their access to CFBs (cigars-for-blunts). This might explain why the inexpensive CFBs remain more popular than blunt wraps for making and smoking blunts.

## Blunt Chasers

Low-cost cigars and blunt wraps used to construct blunts are not the only tobacco products that are related to the blunt smoking phenomenon. Through interviews and direct observations with blunt smokers, an emergent smoking practice was identified. "Blunt chasing" is the practice of passing around a cigar, cigarillo, or cigarette immediately after a blunt is smoked. The most common chasers are cigarillos, or small cigars; these are often deeply inhaled and held in the lungs like marijuana smoke. Some popular cigarillo brands in New York include Black and Mild, Hav-a-Tampa, Garcia Vegas, and Tiparillos. Many of these small cigars have a plastic or wooden tip as a mouthpiece. Blunt chasers are shared and passed in circles, and they may be smoked one of two ways. They can be passed directly after the blunt is passed, or they may be passed and smoked after the blunt is finished. Regular sized cigars and cigarettes are less common, but were still observed being used as blunt chasers, especially by white and Asian blunt users.

Blunt chasing serves a number of different functions. The nicotine in the tobacco consumed in the chaser might accentuate the high of the smoked blunt. The blunt chaser can also serve to further mask the smoke of the marijuana burning inside the blunt. One ethnographic observation at an outdoor concert involved youths passing two regular cigars at the same time a blunt was being smoked. Police officers and onlookers at the event had a difficult time discerning which cigar actually contained the marijuana. The blunt-chasing practice is embedded within the marijuana use rituals, and so provides an additional context where the heavy inhalation of tobacco smoke is acceptable and common. In a recent content analysis of substance use in popular music videos (Roberts et al., 2002) researchers were not always able to identify whether a blunt or a cigar was being smoked in many music videos, and were subsequently coded as "unidentified smoke."

## IMPLICATIONS

Many different factors are involved when blunt smokers make choices of tobacco products for blunt smoking. These considerations are both practical and symbolic. Practical considerations include the ease in the blunt making process, the taste the CFB/blunt wrap may provide, and to mask the smell of burning marijuana. Pragmatic considerations have been always been involved in the phenomena of blunt smoking. Blunts provide a way for groups of youth to share small amounts of usually commercial grade marijuana and provides flavor to the smoked product. Blunts help mask the smell of the marijuana and provide a slower burn and larger paper than a traditional marijuana joint. Users can also avoid cumbersome and suspicious marijuana paraphernalia such as rolling papers, pipes, and bongs. Many subcultural and symbolic factors influence blunt smokers decisions for a CFB. Cigars for blunt smoking, like other commercial products, are affected by consumer trends. These trends are connected with larger fads or trends in music and fashion. The subcultural influences of Hip Hop and Rastafarianism were reoccurring themes that emerged among blunt smokers during analysis of ethnographic interview data. Blunts themselves have become iconic symbols for Hip Hop, urban street life, and young marijuana users. The recent trend of flavoring tobacco products for blunts is an obvious attempt by tobacco manufacturers to take advantage of the practical and subcultural influences affecting young consumers choices of CFBs. In this sense CFB/blunt wrap producers are not simply selling a product, but are also selling an image or status associated with their product. In this case the status is not one associated with the rich, but one associated with the inner-city. Tobacco companies have always been image conscious in the marketing of their products; fine tuning tobacco products to expand sales associated with blunt smoking is another recent example.

Blunt users commonly choose a cigar brand for reasons that are varied and seem normalized. Surprisingly, no respondents explicitly articulated reasons that had anything to do with the euphoric effect (the "high") created by the smoked blunt. Most of the responses emphasized practical and conventional reasons for choosing their particular tobacco product for blunt making. Many of the responses sounded like lines from a cigarette advertisement. Excerpts from responses to the question, "What type of cigar do you purchase to make your blunts with?" included: "White Owl, because they are sweet" and "I like the Dutch Masters because it's mild. And you can taste more of the smoke, and it burns slow."

Connolly contends that "the flavoring phenomenon is the intent of the tobacco companies to recover a receding youthful market" (Connolly, 2004). In the case of flavored cigars and blunt wraps, however, it is not about "recovering" a youthful tobacco market, but about maintaining one–and obtaining new initiates. Tobacco companies manufacturing CFBs appear very aware of trends in the larger tobacco markets, as well as what is popular inside marijuana subcultures. Cigars for blunts (CFBs) have always been marketed to youth and minorities, and flavored blunts constitute a more recent development.

There are many market intersections between tobacco and marijuana that are related to the phenomenon of blunt smoking. Low-cost cigars for blunts are sold in most retail locations in New York City near cigarettes and other tobacco products. Indeed, the sale of these CFB products appears common in most stores selling tobacco products. Likewise, some retail marijuana sellers offer cigars with the purchase of their marijuana, and one marijuana selling storefront was observed selling pre-rolled blunts for 10 dollars. Promotional blunt wraps are distributed at Hip Hop concerts and other events where marijuana use is commonplace. Blunt wraps are sold mainly in tobacco/cigar sections of paraphernalia stores or "Headshops," which maintains a blurred line regarding whether wraps should be considered tobacco products or marijuana paraphernalia.

While tobacco, alcohol, and drug researchers have justifiably focused on cigarettes as the tobacco products most likely to be consumed by youth, they need to pay attention to other forms of tobacco consumption by youth. Blunt smoking is one important form of initiation and regular use of tobacco products. While major international tobacco conglomerates that manufacture and market most cigarettes have also been the most common target of tobacco control, companies that manufacture cigars for blunts have slipped under the radar. Tobacco control advocates and researchers have little awareness of the cigar giant, Altadis. With the exception of White Owls, Altadis U.S.A. appears to have a very substantial role and very large market share of the tobacco products (including flavored CFB) used by blunt consumers. Their strategies appear innovative in expanding the initiation to and regular use of tobacco–especially via cigars and cigarillos–among those adolescents and young adults who prefer blunts.[3]

## NOTES

1. Details regarding this survey will be provided in future papers. The proportions given here are based upon 151 respondents who were primarily blunt smokers.

2. All respondents chose code names for staff to use in this project. This white woman clearly chose her code name from Bob Marley, the famous Jamaican reggae singer and marijuana user. Many code names chosen by subjects cited here are typical argot words used in the blunt subculture.

3. Please refer to photos appearing at the end of the following article for further clarification of items discussed in this article.

## REFERENCES

Connolly, G.N. 2004. Sweet and spicy flavors: New brands for minorities and youth. Tobacco Control 211-212.

Golub, A., Johnson, B.D., and Dunlap, E. 2005a. The growth in marijuana use among American youths during the 1990s and the extent of blunt smoking. Journal of Ethnicity in Substance Abuse, 4(3/4): 1-21.

Golub, A., Johnson, B.D., and Dunlap, E. 2005a. Subcultural evolution and substance use. Addiction Research and Theory 13(3): 217-229.

Golub, A., Johnson, B.D., Taylor, A., and Eterno, J. 2004b. Quality-of-life policing: Do offenders get the message? Policing 26(3): 690-707.

Hamid, A. 2002. The ganja complex: Rastafari and marijuana. Lanham, MD: Lexington Books.

Johnson, B.D., Williams, T., Dei, K., and Sanabria, H. 1990. Drug abuse and the inner city: Impact on hard drug users and the community pp. 9-67. in M. Tonry and J.Q. Wilson (Eds.), Drugs and Crime. Chicago: University of Chicago Press. Crime and Justice Series, V. 13.

Johnson, B.D., Golub, A., and Dunlap, E. 2000. The rise and decline of drugs, drug markets, and violence in New York City. pp. 164-206 in A. Blumstein and J. Wallman (Eds.), The Crime Drop in America. New York: Cambridge University Press.

Johnson, B.D., Bardhi, F., Sifaneck, S.F., and Dunlap, E. 2005. Marijuana argot as subculture threads: Social constructions by users in New York City. (June): 1-32.

Roberts, D.F., Christenson, P.G., Henriksen, L., and Bandy, E. 2002. Substance Use in Popular Music Videos. Office of National Drug Control Policy Publication.

Sifaneck, S., and Kaplan, C.D. 1995. Keeping off, stepping on, and stepping off: The steppingstone theory reevaluated in the context of the Dutch cannabis policy. Contemporary Drug Problems 22(3): 513-546.

Sifaneck, S., Kaplan, C.D., Dunlap, E., and Johnson, B.D. 2003. Blunts and blowtjes: Cannabis use practices in two cultural settings and their implications for secondary prevention. Journal of Free Inquiry in Creative Sociology 31(3): 1-11.

Soldz, S., Huyser, D.J., and Dorsey, E. 2003. Youth preferences for cigar brands: Rates of use and characteristics of users. Tobacco Control, 12:155-160.

# Sessions, Cyphers, and Parties: Settings for Informal Social Controls of Blunt Smoking

Eloise Dunlap, PhD
Bruce D. Johnson, PhD
Ellen Benoit, PhD
Stephen J. Sifaneck, PhD

**SUMMARY.** The importance of settings for marijuana use has been widely noted, but the way that informal social controls are organized to moderate the amounts consumed have not been well documented. A major ethnographic study of blunts/marijuana use in New York City observed several hundred marijuana users in group locations and conducted intensive interviews with 92 focal subjects. The vast majority of blunt

Eloise Dunlap, Bruce D. Johnson, Ellen Benoit, and Stephen J. Sifaneck are affiliated with the National Development and Research Institutes, Inc., New York, NY 10010.

The authors acknowledge the many contributions of Flutura Bardhi, Anthony Nguyen, Doris Randolph, and Ricardo Bracho.

This research was funded by the National Institute on Drug Abuse (NIDA–5R01 DA 013690-04) to study blunts/marijuana use patterns, social, economic, and physical contexts where consumption of marijuana occurs, and the marijuana market. Additional support is provided by other projects (R01 DA09056-10, T32 DA07233-21).

The ideas or points of view in this paper do not represent the official position of the U.S. Government, National Institute on Drug Abuse, or National Development and Research Institutes, Inc.

[Haworth co-indexing entry note]: "Sessions, Cyphers, and Parties: Settings for Informal Social Controls of Blunt Smoking" Dunlap, Eloise et al. Co-published simultaneously in *Journal of Ethnicity in Substance Abuse* (The Haworth Press, Inc.) Vol. 4, No. 3/4, 2005, pp. 43-80; and: *The Cultural/Subcultural Contexts of Marijuana Use at the Turn of the Twenty-First Century* (ed: Andrew Golub) The Haworth Press, Inc., 2005, pp. 43-80. Single or multiple copies of this article are available for a fee from The Haworth Document Delivery Service [1-800-HAWORTH, 9:00 a.m. - 5:00 p.m. (EST). E-mail address: docdelivery@haworthpress.com].

smokers preferred to consume in a group setting. Participants identified three group settings in which blunt smoking often occurred–sessions, cyphers, and parties. The analysis identifies various conduct norms, rituals, and behavior patterns associated with each of these settings. Regardless of the setting, group processes encouraged equal sharing of blunts, moderation in consumption, intermission and breaks between smoking episodes, and involvement in non-smoking activities. Blunt smoking groups rarely encouraged high consumption and intoxication from marijuana. *[Article copies available for a fee from The Haworth Document Delivery Service: 1-800-HAWORTH. E-mail address: <docdelivery@haworthpress.com> Website: <http://www.HaworthPress.com> © 2005 by The Haworth Press, Inc. All rights reserved.]*

KEYWORDS. Blunts, marijuana, sessions, cyphers, subcultures, conduct norms

## INTRODUCTION

In this paper we examine the social construction of informal conduct norms that may act to create controlled smoking patterns among a substantial portion of the blunts subculture. A blunt is marijuana wrapped in a cigar shell (generally Dutch Masters, Phillies Blunt, etc.) and smoked. Our analysis focuses upon informal controls and how they may operate in different social settings. We draw from Zinberg and Harding's (1982) and Erich Goode's (1999) theory of set and setting to examine smoking behavior patterns and conduct norms within the blunts sub-culture. We concentrate primarily upon the setting (mainly social) in which blunt users engage in consumption. We identify and focus upon three specific social settings and the informal conduct norms within them: "session," "cypher," and "party."

Special attention is given to what takes place in these settings and how behavior in these settings may operate to limit blunt use. Although conduct norms vary according to each social setting, there are some commonalities across the settings. An overriding interest is to analyze informal social control mechanisms and the ways in which settings are organized so as to moderate consumption. Within group settings people learn rules: instructions in proper use, attitude toward use, and most importantly, that occasional and moderate rather than intensive patterns of blunt consumption predominate.

# BACKGROUND

Marijuana has a long and complex history as a recreational drug in American society (Musto, 1999). It evolved from clandestine hashish clubs that catered to the well to do (Inciardi, 1986) to being mainly consumed by blacks and Mexicans in the 1920s (Musto, 1999). In the 1930s marijuana became a "drug" that was postulated to be extremely dangerous–corrupting youths, having serious negative impact on health (especially mentally), and encouraging deviant behavior, even murder (Inciardi, 1986; Musto, 1999; Earlywine, 2002). Although examinations of marijuana consumption diminished from the research agenda during the crack era, it has emerged as a social problem due to similar claims of past eras–addiction (Coffey et al., 2003; Wagner & Anthony, 2002; Chabrol, Fredaigue, & Callahan, 2000; Poulton et al., 2001; Grant & Pickering, 1998; Chabrol et al., 2002), damaging physically and mentally (Sridhar et al., 1994; Cohen, 1981; Adams & Martin, 1996; Fried, 1995; Johnson et al., 2000; Kalant, 2004); diminished social responsibility (Whitlow et al., 2004), negative effect on psychosocial functioning and psychopathology (Rey, Martin, & Krabman, 2004), inducing teens to drop out of high school (Bray et al., 2000). It will be important to examine more closely how informal social rituals associated with marijuana/blunt use and examine how users may effectively engage in controlled consumption, rather than exhibit patterns of abuse and addiction to marijuana/ blunts.

## *Marijuana Use in America*

Marijuana is the most commonly used illicit drug in the United States. Over 83 million Americans (approximately 37%) 12 years old and over have at least tried it once (National Household Survey on Drug Abuse, 2004). SAMHSA's 2003 Survey on Drug Use and Health estimated that 3.1 million persons aged 12 or older used marijuana on a daily basis (NSDUH, 2003). This widespread use of marijuana requires a closer analysis of use practices to understand why more marijuana users are not dependent or harmed.

Analysis of the conduct norms within the various social settings will suggest how controlled use of marijuana/blunts may occur. Such a discussion may help to untangle factors that may help to understand the regularity of marijuana/blunt use without the negative byproduct of drug dependency or abuse. Few recent studies examine critical factors in the social settings that may impact on controlled marijuana/blunts use or whether and how the conduct norms within these setting may help to socially limit how much marijuana is used. Prior research, much of it conducted in the 1970s, found that marijuana has less potential for dependence than other substances (Grinspoon, Bakalar, & Russo, 2005; Zimmer & Morgan, 1997) in part due to the social settings in which marijuana consumption took place.

Recent investigations indicate that few people are listed as cannabis dependent compared with the large number of marijuana consumers and new initiates. Most users fall somewhere between those who have used within the past year and those who are open to the use of marijuana (see Dunlap, 2004; Dunlap et al., in review). Studies have shown that small percentages of users were at risk of dependence (Anthony et al., 1994; Chen et al., 2004; Coffey et al., 2003); that most respondents who used marijuana did not progress to addiction (Fergusson & Horwood 2000, 2002; Fergusson et al., 2003); and that marijuana has low potential for dependence, if any (Grinspoon, Bakalar, & Russo, 2005; Zimmer & Morgan, 1997). Such findings suggest that a large proportion of consumers may be controlling their use of marijuana/blunts.

The vast majority of users smoke marijuana more or less on a regular basis and are apparently not dependent. Why is it that so many users do not develop dependency and heavy use? The social setting in which consumption takes place may be an important factor. Blunt users prefer to smoke in group settings. An ethnographic examination also found that the majority of marijuana/blunt smokers did not feel that marijuana was addictive (Dunlap et al. in review). They felt that they could stop when they wanted to do so. Some even stopped to continue a social obligation (i.e. school, work). Indeed, a number stopped smoking because they became bored with, tired of, or simply did not desire to continue to smoke. In addition, some individuals stopped smoking marijuana as an indication that they could stop when they wanted to do so (Dunlap et al., in review). Such findings also suggest that blunt consumption leaves the individual with more latitude to consume in a controlled manner.

As in the 1970s and early 1990s, the recent increase in marijuana consumption (SAMHSA, 2003; Golub & Johnson, 2001; Golub et al., 2004) stimulated a renewed interest in marijuana use under the rubric of addiction and concerns about health hazards (Khalsa et al., 2002; Hashibe, Ford, & Zhang, 2002; Taylor & Hall, 2003). Consequently, the majority of studies have tended to focus upon problematic use and users (Poulton et al., 2001; Swift Hall & Teesson, 2001; Coffey et al., 2003; Wagner & Anthony, 2002; Anthony, Warner, & Kessler, 1994; Chabrol, Fredaigue, & Callahan, 2000; Grant & Pickering, 1998;

Chabrol et al., 2002; Fergusson et al., 2004; Johnson & Golub, 2003). A large percentage of these investigations largely neglect to focus upon the variety of consumption patterns that fall between no use and dependency. A number of studies suggest that after first use there is a gradual transition to more regular use; but at any given time, a minority (usually about 10%) of marijuana users meet the criteria for cannabis dependency (Compton et al., 2004; Dennis et al., 2002; SAMHSA, 2003). In fact, the vast majority of marijuana users do not meet criteria for cannabis dependency; so addiction to marijuana is rarely claimed or reported in the scientific literature (except if it is equated with dependency). The findings in this paper suggest that the level of marijuana use is powerfully influenced by where and how people use marijuana/blunts and the conduct norms they follow in such consumption settings. The focus here is not upon the characteristics that differentiate marijuana/ blunt consumers from those who do not use; rather our main interest is in the various settings and how the conduct norms within these settings may enable consumers to moderate their use. To that end, the norms within three social settings for blunt use occur are examined: "sessions," "cyphers," and "parties."

## Theoretical Underpinnings

The issue of why people use marijuana and the effects of marijuana upon the user have been well examined theoretically (Hirschi, 1969; Johnson, 1973, 1980; Gottfredson & Hirschi, 1990; Akers et al., 1979; Akers, 1992, 1998; Becker, 1963, 1967; Kandel 1973, 1974, 1980; Goode, 1999). Factors involved in the controlled use of illicit drug use are most clearly stated by Zinberg (1984; Zinberg & Harding, 1982). Although he listed pharmacology and mind set as important factors in consideration of drug use/abuse, he also saw *setting* as a critical element in drug consumption. Zinberg's main concern was to learn how people controlled their drug use. Like Goode (1999), Zinberg questioned critical definitions and basic assumptions regarding drug use. They both attempted to describe, analyze and explain drug use phenomena; each tried to describe a reality of drug use based upon analysis of what consumers did and the norms they followed. In the critique of accepted definitions of addiction, abuse and dependence, Zinberg and Goode emphasized the social phenomenon of definitions and how socially accepted patterns in groups influence users rather than only the pharmacological drug effects. Yet few systematic studies have examined the social settings in which blunt consumption takes place. Both Zinberg and Goode, however, regard the social setting as a critical element in drug use patterns. Both see setting as the social and physical environment in which drug use takes place and influence the conduct norms and behavior patterns of users.

Goode stipulates that setting could be a living room in someone's home or a broader social and cultural scene in which drug use takes place. Setting takes into account whether one takes drugs with friends or with strangers. It also involves whether one engages in social activities that may be compatible or incompatible with drug use/abuse. "The context within which drugs are taken influences what one expects and how one feels about the drug-taking experience and, hence, the effects a drug has" (Goode, 1999: 41). Alongside the pharmacological impact of a drug on the individual, he distinguishes "drug effects," which recognizes a broader set of factors. These include "non-specific" factors such as setting, or "the social, physical and legal context in which drug use takes place." This also means that "the social and cultural norms determine how drugs are used and in what quantity and under what circumstances" (Goode, 1999: 30) and even the way the sensations of physiological response are interpreted and socially constructed by users.

"Studies of drug consumption, which burgeoned during the 1960s, tended to equate use (any type of use) with abuse and seldom took occasional or moderate use into account as a viable pattern" (Zinberg, 1984: 3)–a pattern that continues to the 2000s. For Zinberg, the setting constitutes a very important and immediate present influence on drug consumption by an individual, and is especially important for controlling use. The social group influences each individual because the group develops its own social expectations and constructions about the drug. Groups develop their own rituals and sanctions, which are experienced as very real by the individual user. These patterns constitute the main elements of what Zinberg calls informal social control. These are based upon conduct norms which effectively govern the ways marijuana/ blunts is consumed in the following settings. Since the peer group is extremely important in constructing norms (informal rules) for these settings, a rich array of rituals and subtle sanctions are implied. The peer group provides information needed in case of any bad experience, instructions about how much to smoke while present. The group may be sufficiently important that a modest threat of exclusion from the group might be experienced as a sanction.

Although Zinberg (1984) posited three determinants (drug, set and setting) that must be considered in an attempt to understand illicit drug use and the effect of the drug on the user, the critical element of his theory–as with Goode–for this analysis is the various social settings where consumption takes place. While this includes the physical space, it is especially the social environment within which marijuana/blunt use occurs that is most relevant herein. In the social setting, individuals learn (Bandura, 1977) and become acquainted with values and rules of conduct (or conduct norms) that suggest the expected behavior. Conduct norms are group constructions that provide expectations about how a drug should be used, when and where it should be used. In addition, such conduct norms often exist as vague and poorly defined punishments and rewards, what Zinberg referred to as sanctions (also see Golub, Johnson, & Dunlap, 2005)–examples are provided below. Several conduct norms are often organized into stable behavior patterns, often called rituals. These rituals include how the marijuana is acquired, how it is used, the place of use and the activities that take place during and after use of the drug. Rituals have the effect of supporting compliance with conduct norms, and may also enforce sanctions including ways of preventing unwanted drug effects. These conduct norms, rituals and social sanctions may be socially constructed so as to apply different social contexts that range from small discrete clusters of users, i.e., cyphers, through larger collections of users at sessions and parties.

## *METHODS*

Data for this paper comes from an ongoing longitudinal ethnography (5 years) entitled Marijuana/Blunts: Use, Subcultures, and Markets. The same respondents are followed over the period of investigation and participate in both interviews and observation of their marijuana/blunts use. All interviews are tape recorded so that ethnographers can pay close attention to the accounts being told and prompt subjects to provide the most information. Ethnographers first spent time developing a deep level of rapport with respondents. The respondents learned that the ethnographer was interested in learning about their world of blunt/marijuana consumption and was not the police or an undercover agent. Thus, respondents were more likely to give honest and true responses to questions and inquiries. Second, ethnographers sought to "hang out" with respondents so as to directly observe their marijuana/blunt consumption, to learn and experience the conduct norms and behavior patterns followed, in order to understand the rules, rituals, informal controls, and to observe how such consumption fit into daily lives. Project staff seeks to better understand the subculture of blunts and gained an inroad into consumption locations, but without raising suspicion among persons involved in blunts use. Individual subjects and their associates were directly observed in their natural settings so that the conduct norms could be inferred from direct observation as well as by responses to interviews (Glaser & Strauss, 1967).

In addition to the focal subjects, ethnographers also attended numerous parties, clubs, bars, and various gatherings where marijuana/blunts, tobacco, alcohol, and other drugs were used. Ethnographers wrote extensive field notes that were based upon observations of interactions among several hundred persons who were not focal subjects, especially regarding consumption of blunts or marijuana in group settings (Carini, 1975). The ethnographic field notes written by project staff based upon direct observations of blunt users in the various group settings constitute a major source of data cited below.

Respondents between the ages of 15 and 35 were recruited to participate as focal subjects in this investigation. Such subjects were chosen to represent the varied experiences of marijuana joints users and blunt users of varied age, race/ethnicity, gender, and class/neighborhood. We sought individuals who identified with the different subcultures, who were raised and hung out in different locations, and who were from various ethnic backgrounds in order to diversify the ethnographic sample. In order to gain access to the various groups of marijuana/blunt consumers, we hired ethnographers who are demographically diverse (in terms of age, race, gender).

Respondents were recruited from uptown and downtown neighborhoods of Manhattan (Harlem, Lower East Side) in New York City. These two general areas constituted suitable neighborhoods to acquire a sample that was ethnically and economically diverse. Harlem is basically African-American and Latino. The larger Lower East Side (East Village and Chinatown) mainly encompasses residents who are White, Latino and Asian.

The recruitment process involved participant observation, direct observation and informants. The latter contacts were extremely important in gaining initial access to parties and other social gatherings where marijuana/blunts consumption took place. They were also important in arranging introductions to various persons who were involved with blunts or marijuana (see Dunlap & Johnson, 1999). This enhanced acquiring a sample that was diverse in terms of population characteristics and experiences with blunt/marijuana consumption.

Ethnographers recruited marijuana and/or blunt-using subjects who were artists, musicians, college and high school students, inner-city youths, skateboarders, graffiti writers, participants in the club and nightlife scene, computer and technical types, drug dealers, basketball players, and various types of young working professionals who used. Respondents were also chosen to include not only different backgrounds, economic categories, ethnic/racial categories and subcultures but also various experiences. Parental consent was obtained for persons under the age of 18 years old.

A broad range of marijuana/blunts use, patterns, activities, practices, and rituals were included. Compulsive smokers, self-regulated users, and occasional or sporadic (e.g., once a month) users were included, to acquire the full range of consumption behaviors. Respondents reported preferences for consuming marijuana in a variety of modes: blunts, bongs, joints, bubblers, apples, soda cans, one-hitters and vaporizers, and eaten in brownies, cookies, or popcorn. Some expressed preferences in terms of how they smoked, many preferred blunts, while others favored pipes or joints.

Initially 120 respondents of different races, ages, and genders were interviewed. From these, 92 respondents were chosen as focal subjects who would be followed ethnographically for 3-4 years. Their demographic characteristics are shown in Table 1. Males were somewhat more common than female. Ethnicities of focal subjects were quite mixed, but relatively balanced, with nearly a sixth being from Asian/Indian backgrounds. Subjects were young, with 45% under 21. Almost all were single (never married), and represented a wide range of educational backgrounds (data not presented).

These focal subjects completed an in-depth baseline interview and follow-up interviews every 6 months. Three interview schedules were used: screening schedule, baseline schedule, and follow-up interview schedule. The screening schedule helped ensure the desired diversity

TABLE 1. Demographics of 92 Focal Respondents in Ethnographic Study

| Gender | Male | 58% | Age | 14-17 | 22% |
|---|---|---|---|---|---|
| | Female | 42 | | 18-20 | 23 |
| Ethnicity* | White | 35% | | 21-24 | 14 |
| | Black | 29 | | 25-29 | 20 |
| | Latino | 20 | | 30 & Up | 21 |
| | Asian/Indian | 16 | | | |

*Over a quarter of respondents claimed additional ethnic identities to those given.

according to ethnicity, age, gender, and marijuana or blunts experience. The in-depth baseline interview schedule encompassed a number of significant areas of investigation. The intent was to measure the current and past use of marijuana/blunts, alcohol, tobacco, and other illegal drugs; social behavior within markets for marijuana and tobacco; and subcultural conduct norms and contexts for marijuana/blunt use. The baseline interview schedule obtained life-histories from respondents, including life experiences growing up, family life, neighborhood environments, and family member's use of marijuana, other drugs and alcohol. Present day issues regarding lifestyle, subcultural influences, sexual behaviors, and potential criminal and violent behaviors were also explored. The follow-up interview focused on changes in the respondent's use of marijuana, tobacco, alcohol and other drugs, and changes in the subject's life over the last six months.

An important analytical construction was carefully measured in the interview schedules: the distinction between using marijuana primarily in a joint, pipe, or bong and primarily used as a blunt. This distinction between "marijuana" smoked without tobacco and "blunts" was useful on a number of levels. A long range goal of this project is whether use patterns, social rituals, and signs of dependency would differ between respondents who preferred marijuana "joints" and users who primarily smoked marijuana as blunts. This distinction in preferred form of marijuana consumption is reflected in the various social settings and normative aspects of such consumption as reported below. The main focus of this article is upon the social settings associated with blunts consumption, and less so with joint smoking.

## FINDINGS

During the initial interview, respondents were asked, "Do you smoke blunts in a group or alone?" and "Why?" Responses indicated that consumption within a social group is an especially important conduct norm among blunt smokers. Indeed it may be the most prominent: The overwhelming majority (89%) of those who smoked blunts preferred to smoke in groups; very few (4%) preferred smoking blunts alone. Blunt smoking alone is also influenced by the conduct norms found in group settings. The few individuals who reported smoking blunts alone indicated that they usually took a few inhalations and then put the blunt out, thus spacing their consumption during the day–effectively replicating the conduct norms, rituals, and behavior patterns found in the group settings as described below.

The following excerpts indicate conduct norms of group consumption among blunt smokers:

*Tiesha (female, 17 yrs. old, Trinidad):* In a group. Because I don't wanna smoke by myself. I need my friends to be there when I'm smoking just in case something happens to me. You could be hallucinating and stuff and they will know about it. [Ever Tried It Alone?] No.

*Silent Bob (male, 14 yrs. old, Puerto Rican):* In a group because if I get high I don't know what I might do to myself. Yeah safety.

*Tanya (female, 14 yrs. old, Guyana):* It's more fun like that. And, um when I smoke in a group, we share. So, it's so I get high but not to a extreme where I think it's dangerous for me; I just get the right amount when I share.

Additional findings presented below examine the norms found in the different group settings.

### Group Social Settings

Schensul et al. (2000) briefly discussed the social settings in which blunt consumption occurs. Cyphers and sessions were mentioned as equivalent settings for ritual use of blunts. Yet ethnographer observations suggested that these two settings had important differences in their norms and rituals. In addition, respondents in our study reported that these two settings were organized differently.

Three social settings in which blunt consumption typically takes place were called: (1) *sessions*, (2) *cyphers*, and (3) *parties*. These three terms will be employed as analytical constructs to ascertain similarities and differences in the conduct norms and rituals associated with blunts consumption. "Session," "cypher," and "party" can be considered as ideal types and by which to examine the social phenomenon of blunt consumption. Each of these terms is a quick summary word that emphasizes inter-related conduct norms and ritual practices as well as expectations about how many participants of various types are likely to be present. The social relationships embodied in these ideal types are built upon the probability that people will engage in expected actions. These types do not necessarily correspond to concrete reality, but they have been constructed from many ethnographic observations and quotes from transcripts. These types were articulated by respondents and observed by ethnographers. The data from these blunt settings enabled analysts to infer the associated conduct norms, ritual practices, and behavior patterns which may enhance the controlled consumption of blunts Although the settings may be analytically distinguished, they have elements in common, often overlap in actual physical and social locations, and are not mutually exclusive.

Briefly, a "session" occurs when three or more people get together in a designated place to smoke blunts. It is a planned event. In such settings, group norms carry a great deal of weight, and being omitted from the group may be an important sanction. One meaning of a "cypher" is that the group is small and informal, assembles and dissolves, and the gathering is relatively spontaneous. A "party" is a formal gathering in which alcohol is the main substance consumed; blunt smoking takes place where subgroups get together in a separate area from the main social event. In all three settings a variety of informal social controls emerge from the ways in which the settings are organized. What takes place in each setting, the norms, rituals, and behavior patterns followed appear to be very important in moderating blunt consumption. Although a number of conduct norms will be examined in all three settings, two important conduct norms stand out in each. Typical participants: (1) self-select themselves to smoke from available blunts, and (2) share blunts about equally. But these two sharing norms also mask an implicit sanction of disapproval against heavy use and over intoxication. These general conduct norms govern blunt consuming behavior across all three social settings.

## Session

A "session" had several implicit meanings and a variety of conduct norms and rituals. A "session" occurs when a group of people gets together to share in buying, rolling, and smoking blunts. There are five basic characteristics of a session: (1) participants *share* the purchase and *use* of a blunt (marijuana and cigar); (2) it is a planned *indoor* event (generally takes place inside an apartment/club/home/room); (3) generally groups range from small to large, but always involve at least *three people*; (4) they are *long in duration* (people spend time together smoking and participating in some activity); and (5) they usually involve *non-smoking activities* (such as watching a game, movies, dancing, talking, playing cards, etc.).

In a session, people meet specifically to smoke shared blunt(s). The number of people varies depending on the event but it generally consists of more than three, both male and female. In a session, each person puts money in the "bank"[1] to purchase the marijuana and Backwoods, Dutch Masters or Phillies Cigars. Generally $50 is raised, although the amount varies depending on the number of people in the group and the amount of money each individual has to contribute. The expectation is that each person puts up about $10.00, but what one has is acceptable.

Once the money is raised, two people will go to purchase what is needed. One person will go to purchase the "trees" (marijuana) and the other to get the cigars. The individuals making the purchase depends on several factors. An individual who knows a marijuana seller will go to purchase the "trees" because s/he will possibly obtain more product than could usually be bought with the amount of money collected (getting a regular customer discount). The individual who makes the marijuana purchase is often the person who organizes the session, functions as the "banker," or has an apartment where the session will take place. These procedures (rituals) ordinarily take place in sessions: the collection of monies and the sharing of knowledge and expertise; trust that individuals will perform roles expected of them (i.e., purchase marijuana and cigars and return). Sessions may also arise when several friends are together, have enough money, and decide to smoke blunts.

The following quotes from typical respondents indicate how typical consumers understand the importance of the group rituals that occur in blunt sessions:

> *Jay (male, 17 yrs. old, black):* In a group. Like four or five people. Because everybody contribute they money into the smoke so it be more blunts. [why smoke in group] It be more fun. Like when we get high, everybody be laughing and joking and all that.

> *Marley-one (female, 28 yrs. old, white):* Definitely in a group. That's totally a group activity. The whole style of rolling it, breaking, somebody's breaking it up; somebody brought the cigar. Somebody brought the weed. Making sure that, you know, it's good, like for it to take some time, everyone's gonna hang out, sit together. Wait for it to go around, and then go ahead and start whatever social activity we're gonna do.

*Gemi (a 19-year-old Japanese male):* In a group. With blunts, though, it's a different thing. A blunt is more communal. Um, I think it's a collective tradition, like someone buys a Dutch or Phillie, you know what I mean. You know, um, and pass the blunt. You pass the "L" around and it's a lot, you know. The volume of it, the tradition. Um, no. The quantity of it is too much, money wasted on it.

The following excerpt further demonstrates the behavior patterns and conduct norms that minimize specific obstacles youths may encounter. Stores will not sell cigarettes or cigars to youths under the age of 18 years old. Thus youths who smoke blunts and are between the ages of 12 and 17 must have some older person to purchase the shell (cigar) in which to roll the blunt. Someone must have a connection to acquire marijuana and someone must be of age to purchase the cigar. One can have knowledge of one without being able to fulfill the other. The following excerpt from Jalisa, a 14-year-old female Dominican, highlights this aspect of session norms and behavior patterns:

*Interviewer:* Okay. Do you smoke blunts in a group or alone?

*Jalisa:* A group.

*Interviewer:* Why?

*Jalisa:* Because they can get the blunt, but I can't.

*Interviewer:* Others get the cigar?

*Jalisa:* Yeah.

*Interviewer:* They can get the cigar. Okay. Who gets the weed?

*Jalisa:* I could. Yeah, I go get it.

*Interviewer:* Okay. So, you can buy weed.

*Jalisa:* Yeah.

*Interviewer:* Okay. That's funny you can buy weed, but stores, some of the stores won't [sell you a cigar]? . . . Have you ever tried to buy a cigar?

*Jalisa:* Yeah.

*Interviewer:* And they turned you down?

*Jalisa:* Yeah.

This excerpt and the next ones suggest that the group serves a number of purposes for young blunt smokers. In addition sharing the purchase and consumption of the blunt, there is also the drug connection and the shared expertise of participants. This sharing of expertise also includes skill in rolling the blunt:

> *Candy (female, 21 yrs. old, black):* In a group. Four or five people. Usually because other people know how to make blunts. Me, I don't do it by myself. It usually just turns out that way.

> *Aer (male, 16 yrs. old, white):* In a group usually. Well, I don't really know how to roll blunts so it's always usually in a group.

In a session, a conduct norm holds that other activities will take place in addition to smoking the blunt. Individuals expect to smoke, talk, laugh, joke, and often play music, video games, or watch a movie, etc. A session is long in duration and is generally a planned event. If an acquaintance comes by, the blunts are shared even though that person has not contributed money. While rolled blunts may be open in a public place where they can be lit and passed around, the conduct norms effectively stipulate who can light a new blunt and begin to pass it around. Any of the contributors may do this, but not incoming persons (who contributed no money). Rules of conduct also indicate that one individual cannot hold a blunt and smoke the entire joint without passing it to others.

What takes place in a session further suggests the integrative function of blunt smoking (Johnson et al., 2005). Subjects report the closeness of the group and enjoyment of being with friends. This also highlights the theme of trust and camaraderie as values and important source of informal social control. It also suggests that isolation from the group would be painful.

> *Tom (male, 17 yrs. old, black):* A group. Because I just like to be with my people when I'm smoking. [We] Talk. About whatever is on your mind. We talk about everything whatever is on your mind.

We talk about personal stuff like what is going on in people's life or whatever.

*J. Bravo (male, 17 yrs. old, white):* In a group. It makes you have like you get with your friends and ya'll are all laughing and giggling at each other. Ya'll all love the time you're spending together because you're laughing and that's all great to see everybody laughing and having fun knowing they ain't gotta worry about nothing.

*Polo Sparks (male 15 yrs. old, Filipino):* In a group, because then it, it brings unity. Like say if you might have a problem with somebody, but when they smoke, and if you smoke, and say smoking is a different topic within everything else, you can smoke, you could smoke with like your enemy; but you know, like it brings unity. Because people are together and then we smoke in a group.

These excerpts suggest the variety of conduct norms behavior patterns, values, and rituals that are consistent with Zinberg's theory of informal social control. Zinberg emphasizes the importance of social rewards and sanctions about whether and how a particular drug should be used, including informal values, which are generally unspoken, and rules of conduct shared among the group.

Participation in group sessions is voluntary and is here considered as informal interaction. Instructions are passed in an informal manner and are reinforced in such a manner (Zinberg, 1984). Tom, J. Bravo, and Polo Sparks express these informal values by showing how important the group is to the individual. One is free to openly talk about "personal stuff" safely. When individuals are with the group, they feel safe as indicated by J. Bravo: "ain't gotta worry about nothing." Being in the group brings people "together," it "brings unity." These excerpts highlight the importance to its individual members as a collective group. What the group does, each member does.

Physical fights and verbal arguments rarely occurred. In fact, during the years of study (3 years to date), ethnographers seldom observed a physical or verbal fight among blunt consumers during their smoking episodes (Johnson, Golub, & Dunlap, 2000). This suggests that the conduct norms and rituals in blunt-using groups are also intolerant of and discourage violence or threatening actions during smoking episodes–even when some members share some personal animosity toward each other. Polo Sparks demonstrates this when he talks about having an enemy outside the group but when in the group, you smoke with "your enemy" as it brings "unity." While a person may be considered an enemy outside the group, that person cannot be treated as an enemy because the norms of the group do not support antagonistic relationships during a session. These examples demonstrate rules of conduct and how they are informally learned. They also indicate how informal rules set the agenda for how people are to interact in the group setting.

When smoking, one learns what to do by watching what other group members do. When the blunt is passed and the individual sees that everyone only takes one or two puffs from the blunt and then passes it to the next person, so that the "puff-puff-pass" norm becomes an operational rule in the group. In this way, the group provides instruction and reinforces its norms and expectations in an informal manner. The source of precepts and practices and social learning about the drug, how to address the impact of the drug on a person, advice to friends on what to do in certain situations, rituals and sanctions (Johnson et al., 2005) prescribed by the blunt subculture, all occur within the group (Zinberg, 1984; Zinberg & Robertson, 1972).

The following places are the type of social environments in which sessions take place. The first three–apartment/loft, a blunt smoker's apartment, and a rapper's apartment–are intended only to reveal the different environments and to demonstrate how each may reflect the variety of social settings in which sessions may occur. The fourth environment, "session at inner-city apartment," reveals what a session looks like and suggests the rituals, behaviors, norms and experiences in a session.

A "session" takes place in someone's house or inside a closed environment. These apartments range from working to upper middle class homes, tenements to condos, with single adults to families dwelling in them. These locations have been for the most part clean and well-appointed (but not always). The following field notes describe the various environments in which a session takes place.

*Apartment/Loft:* The loft space was artist housing, and was on the second floor. Dave's place had about 4,500 square feet. The building was bombed with graffiti so that the building number was barely legible because it had been painted over. Like many loft spaces in Brooklyn, there was no buzzer so it was necessary to bang on the door to get attention. The apartment was in the process of being renovated. The rooms were built with drywall, which is typical of loft spaces. The walls were covered with graffiti tag names. The floors were raw plywood without carpeting. The most interesting part of the apartment was the bathroom. It had an enormous steel door generally found as the door to a walk-in cooler in restaurants. It was quite creative.

*A Blunt Smoker's Apartment:* I enter her spacious two-bedroom apartment into a large kitchen, The living room has a mod feel, with a white shag rug and two large round orange hanging lamps. A framed and autographed poster of "Andre the Giant has a posse" is one of Susana's most prized possessions. A comfortable white recliner, steel coffee table with long thin legs and a single steel ashtray also occupy the room.

*A Rapper's Apartment:* The apartment is located in the basement. It has two small bedrooms. The kitchen is fairly large with a counter separating the kitchen from the living/dining room. The glass kitchen table has three well worn chairs. The living room has an entertainment center with a television and various electronic gadgets. Three futons line the living room, along with an old well-worn leather chair. The apartment is not well kept; dirty dishes are in the sink, and a portable washing machine is hooked up to the kitchen sink.

These environments reflect the range of places in which blunt sessions were observed. The following field notes give a picture of a large smoking session.

*Session at Inner-City Apartment:* When I entered the apartment, several males were in the room. They had been out drumming all day and had recently come in from this "work." Thomas was a tall lean male around 25 years old who is an excellent rapper. He has recorded some of his rap music and is trying to get it played on the radio. He goes out drumming with his friends to make money because he is unemployed. Kennedy is a professional drummer who plays at functions for his organization of African-American Israelites. Ray is a cousin of Kennedy. Thomas and Kennedy drum on the subway to make money to help them reach a perceived goal (They are trying to get into the music business). Other young males present are ages 24-27. Kennedy, the lead drummer, counts the money, and gives each drummer his share of the money.

Once they split the money, they talk about having a session.

Each contributes $10 except for two, who each contribute $5. Thomas calls a dealer who delivers the marijuana. Ray and his girlfriend go to the store to buy (chocolate) Backwoods cigars. As they wait for the marijuana to arrive Thomas and George play a game. Kennedy makes a call. Everyone sits in a relaxed manner talking about their experiences while drumming. Ray and Sammy get a little concerned that it is taking a long time. The marijuana delivery man arrives about half an hour later. He delivers a medium ziplock bag of brownish-colored marijuana. The Backwoods, beer and cigarettes arrive soon. The bag of marijuana is placed on the table and Thomas and Kennedy begin to roll blunts. Each rolls about two blunts (total 4) and places them on the table. Once they roll the blunt they light one and pass it around. The blunt is held for a short span of time before it is passed to the next person. Approximately three puffs are taken and it is then passed. Everyone has come closer together, sitting on the futons or standing. As they smoke they also talk, joke, and laugh. They also drink the beer and smoke cigarettes. After finishing a blunt they take break. Various activities occur with intermissions between smoking episodes.

During this time, additional people come to the apartment and more blunts are lit and begin to go around the room. At one point I counted three blunts being passed around at one time. During this time every one continued to socialize, take a few puffs from the blunt, pass it and maintain what they were doing such as laughing, talking, playing games and simply standing around. At one point Thomas began to "rap" to show new verses he had made up. This session lasted for at least 4 hours before I left and was still taking place with people coming and going.

These field notes and interview excerpts reveal two main aspects of setting: rituals and sanctions. These rituals and sanctions may suggest control over consumption. First, the norm of taking a few puffs before passing the blunt suggest that individuals must be able to control their consumption at specific points in time. They cannot continue to smoke the blunt without passing it to others. In addition, blunts are not constantly smoked; rather, there are several points of intermission in which people stop blunt use. Further, some members who reached their desired "high," decline their turn when the blunt comes to them. This also suggests a conduct norm against being highly inebriated during a session. Furthermore, what began as a session (with five persons present) to smoke blunts, began to resemble a party (see below) as several additional persons stopped by to participate in both drinking alcohol and smoking blunts.

## Cypher

A "cypher" is quite different from a session in the number who participate, the duration, and the purpose of the group. The fundamental conduct norm in a cypher is to get high quickly. Sharing is limited to a few participants. When cyphers occur outdoors, a concern is not to draw attention. The primary purpose of a cypher is to smoke, acquire the high, and then disperse. A cypher can start with as little as one person sitting on a park bench smoking a blunt and a friend walks by and is invited to share the blunt. Or two persons, one has an "L" (a blunt) and a friend joins in smoking. A cypher may also occur when a small group of persons go off from a larger group to smoke.

> *John Doe (male, 15 yrs. old, black):* If Mark has one, they, Jimmy has one and it's just me, I might as well go get one. If I want to smoke too, I'm gonna get one.

> *How High (male, 30 yrs. old, Jamaican):* If I'm like walking down the block and I have it or they [friends] have weed or whatever or if I had a blunt and I was walking and they asked me I might just chill with them and what not.

A cypher actually occurs, as does the session, in many different forms. Unlike a session, a cypher is not formed with a plan to buy marijuana, rather someone already has it. A cypher often occurs when individuals do not have a private or inside place to smoke, so it usually occurs outside, in public space–but it does not have to take place outside. A cypher has central characteristics: a few persons gather inconspicuously to smoke, usually outdoors; it is generally spontaneous (not previously planned); it takes place in a shorter amount of time; there are few non-smoking activities; it involves a small group of persons, and can not grow too big in number. Unlike a session or a party, a newcomer to a cypher is expected to provide (a conduct norm) a blunt to add to what is being passed around. An individual can not walk into a cypher and expect to share the common blunt (a social sanction), unless a current participant invites them to take part. During a cypher, participants may be relatively quiet, or have ordinary conversations while smoking.

Conversations in cyphers are not long; rather talk is brief, polite and often focused upon the blunt smoking.

The conduct norms and ritual associated with cyphers differ from those of a session in the following respects: (1) usually one or more participants already have marijuana and/or a rolled blunt; (2) participants don't have to collect money and/or collectively purchase the marijuana, (3) participants generally must be invited into the cypher, (4) but having a blunt to share will gain an invitation; (5) finally, participants share the blunt(s) equally (puff-puff-pass), (6) they get moderately high; (7) when the blunt(s) is finished, the group dissolves or goes off to do something else.

## Cypher Settings

This section examines the various type of settings in which cyphers occur. Field notes depict what takes place. Cyphers are less organized than a session and informal social control is diffused.

> *Club/Bar Setting as Cypher:* I arrived at Lola's, a bar in the Lower East Side of Manhattan at about 10:30 PM on a busy Friday night. The DJ was spinning new wave and 1980s classics. He had black spiky hair that was feathered and dressed in all black.
>
> Since the [NYC] anti-smoking law is in effect, many people went outside the bar to have a cigarette and–as I later found out–to smoke marijuana/blunts. Although it was cold outside, many people were outside smoking cigarettes. Like a social club, smokers stick together in a smoke-free world.
>
> Two friends of a friend of mine showed. One was Asian with short straight black hair and the other was white, about 5'10", with dark brown hair that was short and shaggy. Both work for a high-end marijuana delivery service based out of Manhattan; they had just gotten off of work. Since there were a lot of smokers outside the bar, they decided to smoke a blunt. The Asian took out a blunt that he had rolled earlier out of his sweatshirt pocket. It was rolled with Backwoods, and when he lit it and passed it to his friend, I could smell the familiar sweet vanilla tobacco scent that Backwoods emanates.
>
> The blunt went around in a circle and everyone took a long hit off of it. It was incredible to watch this scene go down, right outside the front door of a bar that has enormous glass windows. Ev-

eryone continued to smoke the blunt, passing it around time and time again, and often sneaking in a puff of a cigarette in between.

No one walked by as this puff-fest was taking place, and no one came in or out of the bar. After they completed smoking, everyone piled back into the bar at once, sitting down and hanging out together. It was like a little clique of the smokers vs. the non-smokers. Anytime someone wanted to go outside for a smoke, whether it was to smoke cigarettes or pot, a group of three to five people would filter out to join them.

*Empty Lot Cypher:* Ducky (17), Sunny (17), and Wide Eyes (18) are all Chinese-American males who reside where Chinatown meets the Lower East Side. I met them at a game room. Sunny, Ducky and Wide Eyes showed up at the game room about 25 minutes late. They motion for me to come outside. It seemed they did not want to make a big scene inside the game room about knowing me, after all I was much older, white, and could possibly be a cop. They greeted me in sort of a "I'm cooler than you" manner shaking my hand in the customary three step "street" shake. We proceeded about 50 feet down the block into an empty lot.

Ducky took out a Vanilla Dutch Masters cigar, a Hip Hop magazine, and what appeared to be 1/8 of an ounce of high quality hydroponics marijuana. "This is some nice shit, yo, just bought it" he boasts. He then told me he paid $35 for 1/8 of an ounce (3.5 grams) of "hydro" from downtown Chinese weed delivery service. I note that this price is far less than what most of our white respondents pay for similar quality stuff. Ducky then places about 1 gram of the marijuana into the empty Dutch Masters cigar shell. This is a relatively large amount of high quality material for a blunt for three people, but the group gives the impression that marijuana comes and goes easily. As Ducky finishes rolling the blunt Wide Eyes and Sunny are watching, and getting antsy with anticipation.

I ask Sunny why they call this a "Cypher" and he explains that's what people consider assembling in a circle in order to pass a blunt around. Cypher may be a term that evolved out of the phenomenon of "Freestyling" in Hip Hop. This is where rappers would assemble in a circle and make up spontaneous rhymes that would be shared with people in the circle. What I was observing was certainly a small cypher since it only consisted of three people. Each person took an average of three pulls off the blunt at each pass, and talking in between pulls was not uncommon. While they were smoking a police cruiser passes by, but the group is not fully visible since the lot is off-set from the street. We however can see the cruiser in full view. I ask whether they should be concerned and Wide Eyes replies with a grin, "they don't worry about us, we don't worry about them." Their reactions gave me the impression that their interactions with the police are very limited.

As the blunt was passed there was some conversation, but that was limited to short interactions often supplemented by hand and facial gestures. It seemed these three men had a definite intent: roll a blunt, smoke a blunt, get high, and then get back to playing games at the video parlor. Conversation was limited during the cypher because the focus was on getting high in an outdoor public place and getting back to other activities. The conversation that did take place was also limited to topics that the three had already been discussing earlier in the day: a recent basketball game and girls in school. The three finished about 2/3's of the blunt, wrapped it in a piece of a brown paper bag, and put it away (the remainder of their bag of marijuana was not used at that time). The total duration of the cypher was about 12 minutes.

These examples are fairly typical because the cyphers took place outdoors. Especially in a cypher, users and non-users may be together in the same social context (a bar or game room here). Generally users separate themselves from the non-users by going outdoors and find a space away from the non-users. Use does not take place in the entire environment, but only in a small group setting within the larger environment. Small groups are where the social control occurs. Although users do not go out of their way to conceal their blunt use, they appear to follow conduct norms of respecting non-smokers' environment; so the blunt and tobacco smokers separate from the larger group and/or go outside to indulge. In both cyphers above, consumers may not smoke the entire blunt, and may even put it out if they are high enough for the time being. Users then do something else. But users may also reassemble the cypher (perhaps involving different persons) for smoking another blunt. Thus, several different blunt smoking episodes may occur, but be interspersed with non-smoking activities, several times during an evening. The various rituals and conduct norms are strongly suggestive of informal group-regulated blunt smoking practices that are supportive of getting high or moderately euphoric, but also encourage wide spacing of blunts smoking episodes, effectively avoiding high levels of intoxication and/

or excessive consumption of marijuana. The next setting, "party," contains elements of both the session and the cypher.

*Party*

A "party" is the third setting in which blunt consumption often occurs. A party is a planned gathering in which many people come together to socialize; normally alcohol is served, enthusiastic conversations take place; people stand around talking in large and small groups; dancing may occur, etc. Informal rules, reinforced by New York City anti-smoking regulations, suggest that blunt smokers separate themselves from non-smokers when smoking blunts. Those who do not smoke will continue to enjoy the party and will not pay undue attention nor sanction those who have segregated themselves. Individuals at the party who smoke blunts will usually walk around the party to see whether or where persons may be smoking.

Blunt smokers do not completely separate themselves from others in the party. They may go back and forth socializing with both smokers and non-smokers, except when blunt smoking occurs. A party differs from a "session" and "cypher" in that people do not gather specifically to smoke blunts, more persons use alcohol, and limited sharing of blunts may occur.

A party has specific characteristics that are both similar to and different from the session and the cypher setting. As with a session, a party is pre-planned, it usually takes place indoors, it is a large gathering, long in duration, and involves many non-smoking activities. The owner/host typically provides the physical space and pays for most of the expenses associated with the party. The sharing aspect of a session may be similar in some respects in that sometimes guests contribute by bringing a bottle of wine, liquor, or even a dish of food to a party. In most parties, socializing is the main event and guests stay for a period of time, to talk, dance, listen to music, and so forth. Blunt smoking may be a relatively minor aspect of the event (as in the birthday party), or a central activity (as in the dealer's party) described below. In a party, alcohol is in public view and available to everyone; it is the accepted mode of altered consciousness. Often an assigned person–bartender–provides the drinks, or users may pour their own.

As with sessions, the party follows rituals, informal rules, and values. Those who wish to smoke blunts are expected to separate themselves into another room or location. Typically, any party attendee can feel free to join the small group (like a cypher) and share equally in blunt smoking whether they know one another or not. Those smoking blunts are not expected to contribute money. Nonsmokers at the party do not complain nor attempt to sanction those smoking blunts/marijuana.

Those smoking at a "party" follow many practices that are similar to "cyphers." Individuals voluntarily separate from the larger party, go to a separate room or location (typically a private indoor space), and congregate with the specific purpose of smoking blunts. Unlike cyphers, users at a party do not go outside (in some cases they do), but separate themselves by gathering in a corner of the room or in another room to smoke blunts. The primary purpose is to smoke the blunt, get moderately high, and not necessarily to socialize. Such gatherings may be considered as spontaneous in that users do not plan ahead of time to separate, but do so when they find others smoking blunts. In addition, comparable to a cypher (where numbers are limited), while an initially small group of people gather in the party setting, the number of blunts users can grow much larger than in most cyphers. Although socializing takes place, it is limited while blunt smoking because the main socializing is carried out in the larger party setting. Finally, a party setting also differs from sessions and cyphers, in that many non-users of blunts/marijuana (and often tobacco) are present and socialize with one another.

*Upper Middle Class Birthday Party:* One afternoon, I went to a birthday party of three friends who use blunts (Audrey, Aeryn, and Sunny). I learned that I had not dressed in the formal attire. Audrey is dressed formal attire. It is evident by her attire that the birthday friends have a "Breakfast at Tiffany's" theme. Thus many people are dressed in semi-formal attire. I estimate that there are a good one hundred guests at the party. Guests were congregating in a large, spacious area; a long line could be seen leading to the bathroom. A bartender served mixed drinks behind a makeshift bar. The males are dressed in a J.Crew/Banana Republic style, wearing tucked in collared shirts with khaki pants and leather dress shoes. Almost all have their hair cut short and neatly groomed. Many of the females wear dresses or skirts. The birthday party is in honor of both Aeryn, a 21-year-old Chinese-American student at a major university in New York, and Audrey, who is very interested in the glitzy and glamorous sides of the entertainment industry. A self-described "fag-hag," she also loves to gossip, and has a very bubbly personality.

I asked Aeryn if any of her friends who smoked blunts are at the party, and she told me that most of them are here. I was able to meet many of them. The first person she introduced me to was Sunny, who is the third of the birthday girls. A great deal of drinking and dancing–but no blunt smoking–takes place until around 2 AM at which time many people have left the party. At this time, I notice a small gathering of people in the corner of the room passing around a small joint. They do not seem to be talking much, but more leaning against the walls, couches, or shelves that are located around them. They all have a very relaxed demeanor; I notice that they also all blow their smoke out the window of the apartment, which has been opened very wide. They are not attempting to be discreet about their smoking; it appears they are more enjoying the cool breeze coming into the room. The smell of the marijuana in the air is very faint, but the scent can be distinguished from the tobacco smoke floating in the room.

Later, I notice in a group passing a blunt around the bedroom. It appears that about five people are sharing the blunt. I cannot tell what the blunt has been wrapped in because I do not smell any particular scents that may lead me to believe it had been wrapped in one of the flavored blunt wraps (ethnographer, Asian, male).

*Party at Dealer's Apartment:* Dave is a 23-year-old Korean male who immigrated to the U.S. when he was nine years old. He went through the NYC public school system, graduated high school, and then began selling high quality marijuana. He has been selling to his friends and some people in his neighborhood since he moved into the loft space five months ago. Dave is also a professional photographer and loves to skateboard and snowboard.

Dave, Marie, Roy, Lily and I were sitting at the wooden kitchen table and everyone was drinking and celebrating. Roy and Dave asked if anyone wanted to smoke a blunt, and Marie nodded. Dave pulled a lighter, two Dutch Masters and a plastic zip lock bag with two grams of marijuana out of his pocket. Roy threw down an eighth of marijuana that was tightly vacuum sealed in a small plastic cube and a package of Backwoods onto the table. At that moment another 10 to 15 people walked into the room.

Dave broke up the marijuana, which was green and appeared to be high quality. I could barely smell it. He took a copy of *Vice* magazine (a local Brooklyn magazine about street culture and fashion) that was on the table, opened up the Dutch Master, removed the tobacco and the inner shell, inserted the marijuana into it, rolled it tightly, licked the side of the shell and sealed it. He then lit it and passed it to the left around the table. Roy took a couple of hits and passed it to Marie. Marie took a hit and passed it to a friend of her's who had walked in with the group of people. Hillary then passed it to her friend Ali, and so on and so on.

More and more people started showing up. It was about 10:45 PM at this point. Roy decided to mingle around the room with his blunt. He broke up his marijuana, which was very high quality. The instant he opened up the plastic cube, the smell of it filled the room. It was minty, the same pine tree smell that I had smelled when I interviewed him. He rolled the blunt so quickly and efficiently; he was a pro at it. He then grabbed his beer cup, stuck the blunt in his mouth, lit it, and went to mingle with the guests. Morrie and Mr. X were among the people he went to talk to, and they all smoked the blunt together.

As reflected in these observer notes, a party has some elements of both the session and the cypher. Similar to the session, a party is planned, but is different as the host usually provides almost all the alcohol for all the guests. Guests are not expected to chip in to buy drinks nor blunts. What is also interesting is the different norms regarding blunts use in the two excerpts above. The birthday party had a very large crowd with many (probably) non-marijuana users; socializing, drinking, dancing were the main activities when most persons were present. Only after 2:00 AM did several small groups of blunt smokers begin using in the corners or bedrooms. At the dealer's party, blunt smoking was a primary activity shared by most attendees. Indeed, many attendees were probably occasional customers or users, who got "free" use of high quality marijuana at this party.

> *Monchi (female 26 yrs. old, Cuban-American):* If I were to come across one [blunt] it would definitely be in a group, at a party. Yeah! I see them more like when I used to have parties and stuff like that and there would be a blunt and it would be enough to get like twenty people stoned . . . well, not really but like ten, you know what I mean! It's like a party, it's more social and collective.

This quote implies that parties are also likely to be the main setting in which very intermittent users (and possibly neophytes) are likely to have an opportunity to smoke blunts without being expected to pay for it and/or acquire it. They can smoke "for free" and have no obligation to use it further, nor to participate in such blunt-using groups in the future.

By contrast, such intermittent users are very unlikely to be invited to (and effectively excluded from) a cypher or session.

## DISCUSSION

During this research project involving observations of several hundred blunts/marijuana smoking groups, in both private and public settings, contacts with police or social control agents were rarely observed and/or reported. Thus, legal and formal social controls were rarely observed or reported by focal subjects and user groups. The major factors limiting blunts and marijuana consumption were the social settings described herein.

This paper analyzes three social environments (or group settings) in which blunt consumption often takes place. In each setting, somewhat different conduct norms, values, rituals, and behavior patterns have emerged that have the effective result of controlled consumption of blunts. Informed by Zinberg (1984) and Goode (1999) who stress the importance of the informal controls in various social settings, this analysis focused upon how groups of blunts users may control their consumption and/or limit their dependency upon marijuana. The expectations among group members (that is, the conduct norms) and actual processes associated with consumption (the rituals), result in routines (behavior patterns) that limit the intensity of the blunt smoking experience by most users. The processes in these group settings may be analytically categorized as "active" and "silent." Active processes involve those conduct norms and rituals that guide the activities during blunt-use episodes. Silent processes refers to those conduct norms that systematically limit potential participation in blunt smoking episodes. Examples of both are given below.

*Active controls in group setting.* Several important conduct norms were reported by subjects and routinely observed by ethnographers. Blunt users: (1) expected and wanted to smoke with others in a group setting; (2) expected to contribute money to group purchase(s) of marijuana and cigars; (3) willingly shared the blunt equally among those present; (4) experienced moderate levels of euphoria; (5) typically had intermissions (breaks) between different episodes of blunt smoking; (6) systematically separated from nonusers prior to beginning blunt smoking; and (7) engaged in several other activities (talking, listening, rapping, dancing) before, during, and after blunt/marijuana smoking.

These conduct norms were reinforced by several rituals regarding where, when, and how blunts were consumed–but these varied by setting. Cypher rituals were the least complicated. Usually one or two individuals had previously purchased marijuana and cigars and often initiated sharing it with a few other blunt-using friends. The cypher occurred in a concealed or isolated location, but usually in a public space. It typically lasted a short time (often 15 minutes or less). Participants typically smoked one or two blunts, and reported becoming moderately high–but they rarely became very intoxicated. The group ended that blunt-use episode and dissolved as a group or moved on to other activities. Blunt users who could not contribute marijuana and nonusers were excluded from almost all cyphers. While the same individuals might subsequently resume as a group, initiate another cypher and complete a blunt smoking episode, a break of several minutes to hours had often occurred. Thus, the actual amount of marijuana inhaled by a typical cypher member was limited by the number of blunts involved, the number of participants, and the spacing between consumption episodes. If the marijuana quality was especially good and only a few cypher members were present, a blunt might be "put out" before completion, and saved for later consumption (as in the empty lot cypher).

The rituals associated with blunt smoking during parties were quite similar to cyphers, but participation was less exclusive. Since parties typically involved many persons, often with many non-marijuana users and non-smokers in attendance (as in the birthday party), blunt smokers ritually segregate themselves to a location somewhat removed from the main party (but indoors), and often do so at a late hour. The small groups formed at a party to smoke blunts are likely to be supplied by one or more persons who have brought marijuana and cigars, but without expectation of monetary contributions. While initially only a few persons may join a blunt smoking group at a party, as the blunt is passed around, others at the party may come in and "join" the group. Some persons reported they had mainly discontinued marijuana use, but reported very occasional blunt use at parties or special occasions. So the blunt smoking group may grow relatively larger at a party than at a cypher. Despite contributing no money and not being clearly invited to join, such party members still expect to share (puff-puff-pass) the blunt(s) equally. If too many people smoke, the marijuana supply may run out. So consumption may be limited for all persons present. On the other hand, parties organized by marijuana sellers often include their customers and potential customers, so the supply of marijuana is greater, and blunt smoking is a more central activity than is usually true for parties.

But by controlling the quality of the marijuana and the number of blunts created and circulated, sellers may also limit the amounts consumed by individual participants.

Sessions probably have the most elaborate rituals associated with blunts smoking. Sessions involve relatively systematic organization before use begins. Several blunt users need to agree to meet at a given time and place for the session. In addition, each is expected to bring enough money to make a significant shared contribution to the purchase of marijuana and blunts. Each contributor must trust that the "banker" will not steal or short the money and/or the drugs. [Note: heroin and crack users are much more mistrustful.] The current widespread use of marijuana delivery services–as opposed to marijuana purchases from street sellers–has reduced the likelihood that the banker will take some for his/her own use. Once the marijuana and cigars are obtained, the major monetary contributors often have major roles in rolling the blunts, initiating the lighting of the blunt, and informally monitoring the equal consumption of the blunt by participants. They also determine when to begin another blunt–thus, the spacing between blunt smoking episodes during the session. Blunt smoking sessions tend to last several hours, and have several other activities in addition (talking, laughing, eating, drinking, dancing, acting, games). Most of the persons present at a session will be blunt smokers; they will often be joined by other "friends" who appear to partake for no monetary contribution. Although sessions are organized to purchase relatively large amounts of marijuana, several people may be involved, so that the actual amounts consumed per individual may be relatively modest.

Across cyphers, sessions, and parties, similar rituals and social sanctions operate in the various social contexts: the behavior pattern of smoking small portions and passing the blunt, raising funds and sharing the marijuana, perceiving the group setting as safe, camaraderie among users, taking breaks (spacing) between blunt episodes, and a typically limited supply of marijuana. Following these norms and rituals means that the blunt consumption of most individuals occurs in a controlled manner. The norms and rituals among such groups function as a yardstick and highlight the value of moderation and informal distaste for overindulgence in blunts/marijuana.

*Silent informal controls.* In addition to the active social controls indicated above, many other informal controls operate largely "outside" the blunt-using contexts or group settings, but are effective in reducing the individual opportunities for participation in blunt-using settings. The strong conduct norm for smoking blunts in a group setting, especially when organized as a session, often involves important constraints associated with time, money, and place. That is, motivated blunt smokers must choose among many other activities and commitments (with family or business), agree to attend a session at given date/time, earn/bring enough money to contribute to the bank, actually show up at the session, and have a block of time (often several hours) set aside for blunt smoking. If even one of these conditions is absent (e.g., other commitments on that date, not enough money), individual members would be unlikely to attend the session. At the session, the banker must raise sufficient funds from members, locate a marijuana seller or delivery service, wait for the marijuana purchase to be completed, and trust the purchaser to return with the entire purchase. If the marijuana purchaser becomes unavailable, previously planned blunt sessions would be unlikely to occur or need to be rescheduled. Obtaining the marijuana may be a time consuming activity before blunt smoking rituals begin. In addition, $50 worth of commercial grade marijuana may be enough to create 3-4 blunts, which will likely be equally shared among 4-6 persons. This may provide a modest euphoric effect for each participant, but will be insufficient for the participants to achieve an intoxicated state. There may not be enough money to make additional purchases, or more delay in securing new supplies.

The number of contingencies–especially having enough money and arranging a convenient time/place for each peer group member–is likely to make blunt sessions relatively intermittent affairs rather than highly regular activities for most users. Indeed, except for under- and unemployed groups, most blunt sessions appear to be scheduled as part of recreational days and time (weekends and evenings). Indeed, due to such scheduling difficulties, sessions and parties do not take place every day or even every weekend (Parker, 2005); this limits opportunities an individual may have to smoke blunts.

One potentially important form of informal social control is conspicuously absent or silent. The nonusers of marijuana within a blunt smoker's social networks rarely speak up to clearly state their opposition to such use (Parker, 2005). This is especially evident at party settings when many nonusers effectively ignore groups of blunt smokers. Many blunt users perceive that their non-using friends would not and did not sanction them when smoking. By segregating themselves from nonusers, however, blunt-using groups further reduced the potential of some kind of sanction or disapproval from non-using friends.

Although a modest increase in marijuana/blunt consumption has occurred in the past decade (SAMHSA, 2003; Golub et al., 2004), the findings from this ethnographic study suggest that most blunt smoking occurs in group settings, where the conduct norms and rituals (Zinberg, 1984; Goode, 1999) effectively encourage intermittent use episodes, and moderate rather than intensive consumption. Moreover, the vast majority of blunt use episodes occur in private locations, or are hidden from observation when in public settings. Blunt users report few contacts with police or other formal social control agents, so the informal social controls exerted by group members upon individual users within cyphers, sessions, and parties constitute the major and among the most effective way for limiting consumption by blunt and marijuana users.[2]

## NOTES

1. The bank is the "pot" or pool of money being combined to buy the marijuana and cigars.

2. Please refer to photos following this article for clarification of items discussed in this and preceding article.

## REFERENCES

Adams, I.B., & B.R. Martin. 1996. Cannabis: Pharmacology and toxicology in animals and humans. *Addiction.* 91:1585-1614.

Akers, R.L., M.D. Krone, L. Lanza-Kaduce, & M. Radosevich. 1979. Social learning and deviant behavior: A specific test of a general theory. *American Sociological Review.* 44: 636-655.

Akers, R.L. 1998. *Social Learning and Social Structure: A General Theory of Crime and Deviance.* Boston: Northeastern.

Akers, R.L. 1992. *Drugs, Alcohol, and Society: Social Structure, Process, and Policy.* Belmont, CA: Wadsworth.

Anthony, J.C., L.A. Warner, & R.C. Kessler. 1994. Comparative epidemiology of dependence on tobacco, alcohol, controlled substances, and inhalants: Basic findings from the National Comorbidity Survey. *Experimental and Clinical Psychopharmology,* 2:244-268.

Bandura, A. 1977. *Social Learning Theory.* Englewood Cliffs, NJ: Prentice Hall.

Becker, H.S. 1963. *Outsiders: Studies in the Sociology of Deviance.* New York: Free Press.

Becker, H.S. 1967. History, culture, and subjective experience: An exploration of the social bases of drug-induced experience. *Journal of Health & Social Behavior.* 8: 163-176.

Bray, J.W., G.A. Zarkin, C. Ringwalt, & J.F. Qi. 2000. The relationship between marijuana initiation and dropping out of high school. *Health Economics.* 9(1): 9-18.

Carini, P. 1975. *Observation and Description: An Alternative Methodology for the Investigation of Human Phenomena.* Grand Forks, ND: University of North Dakota Press.

Chabrol, H., N. Fredaigue, & S. Callahan. 2000. Epidemiological study of cannabis abuse and dependence in 256 adolescents. *Encephal.* Jul-Aug 26(4):47-49.

Chabrol, H.E. Massot, A. Montovany, K. Chouicha, & J. Armitage. 2002. Patterns of use, cannabis beliefs and dependence: Study of 159 adolescent users. *Archives of Pediatrics* 9(8):780-788

Chen, K., A.J. Sheth, D.K. Elliott, & A. Yeager. 2004. Prevalence and correlates of past-year substance use, abuse, and dependence in a suburban community sample of high-school students. *Addictive Behaviors.* 29(2): 413-423.

Coffey, C., J.B Carlin, M. Lynskey, L. Ning, & G.C. Patton. 2003. Adolescent precursors of cannabis dependence: Findings from the Victorian Adolescent Health Cohort Study. *The British Journal of Psychiatry.* 182:330-336.

Cohen, S. 1981. Adverse effects of marijuana: Selected issues. *Annals of the New York Academy of Sciences,* 362:119-124.

Compton, W.M., Grant, B.F., Colliver, J.D., Glantz, M.D., & F.S. Stinson. 2004. Prevalence of marijuana use disorders in the United States: 1991-1992 and 2001-2002. *Journal of the American Medical Association,* 291, 2114-2121.

Dennis, M., Babor, T.F., Roebuck, M.C., & Donaldson, J. 2002. Changing the focus: The case for recognizing and treating cannabis use disorders. *Addiction,* 97 (Suppl. 1), 4-15.

Dunlap, E. 2004. Social Construction of Dependency & Addiction by Blunt Users; Ethnographic Reports. Presentation to *College on Problems of Drug Dependency.* June 12-17, San Juan Puerto Rico.

Dunlap, E., E. Benoit, S.J. Sifaneck, & B.D. Johnson. 2005. Social constructions of dependency by blunts smokers: Ethnographic reports. In review.

Earlywine, M. 2002. *Understanding marijuana: A new look at the scientific evidence.* Chapter 1 pp 3-28. New York: Oxford University Press.

Fergusson, D.M., & L.J. Horwood. 2000. Cannabis use and dependence in a New Zealand birth cohort. *New Zealand Medical Journal.* 113, 156-158

Fergusson, D.M., L.J. Horwood, M.T. Lynskey, & P.A.F. Madden. 2003. Early reactions to cannabis predict later dependence. *Archives of General Psychiatry.* 60(10):1033

Fergusson, D.M., L.J. Horwood, & N. Swan-Campbell. 2002. Cannabis use and psychosocial adjustment in adolescence and young adulthood. *Addiction,* 97: 1123-1135.

Fried, P.A. 1995. Prenatal exposure to marihuana and tobacco during infancy, early and middle childhood: Effects and an attempt at synthesis. *Archives of Toxicology Supplement* 17: 233-260.

Glaser, B., & L.L. Strauss. 1967. *The Discovery of Grounded Theory: Strategies for Qualitative Research.* Chicago: Aldine.

Golub, A., & Johnson, B. D. 2001. The rise of marijuana as the drug of choice among youthful arrestees. National Institute of Justice *Research in Brief,* NCJ 187490.

Golub, A., B.D. Johnson, & E. Dunlap. 2005. Subcultural evolution and substance use. *Addiction Research and Theory* 13(3): 217-229.

Golub, A., B. D. Johnson, E. Dunlap, & S.J. Sifaneck. 2004. Projecting and monitoring the life course of the marijuana/blunts generation. *Journal of Drug Issues.* Spring 361-388.

Goode, E. 1999. *Drugs in American Society.* New York: McGraw-Hill Companies.

Gottfredson, M.R., & T. Hirschi.1990. *A General Theory of Crime.* Stanford, CA: Stanford Univ. Press.

Grant, B.F., & R. Pickering. 1998. The relationship between cannabis use and DSM-IV cannabis abuse and dependence: Results from the National Longitudinal Alcohol Epidemiologic Survey. *Journal of Substance Abuse.* 10(3):255-264.

Grinspoon, L., J.B. Bakalar, E. Russo. 2005. Marijuana: Clinical aspects. In J.H. Lowinson, P. Ruiz, R.B. Millman, and J.G. Langrod (Eds), *Substance Abuse: A Comprehensive Textbook,* 4th ed., Baltimore: Williams and Wilkins. 263-276.

Hashibe M., D.E. Ford, & Z.F. Zhang. 2002. Marijuana smoking and head and neck cancer. *Journal of Clinical Pharmacology* 42(11 Suppl):103S-107S.

Hirschi, T. 1969. *Causes of Delinquency.* Berkeley: University of California Press.

Inciardi, J.A. 1986. *The War on Drugs: Heroin, Cocaine, Crime, and Public Policy.* California: Mayfield Publishing Co.

Johnson, B.D. 1973. *Marihuana Users and Drug Subcultures.* New York: John Wiley.

Johnson, B.D. 1980. Toward a theory of drug subcultures pp. 110-119. In *Theories on Drug Abuse: Selected Contemporary Perspectives* (Ed.) by Dan Lettieri. Rockville, MD: National Institute of Drug Abuse.

Johnson, B.D., F. Bardhi, S.J. Sifaneck, & E. Dunlap. 2005. Marijuana argot as subculture threads: Social constructions by users in New York City. *British Journal of Criminology.* June: 1-32.

Johnson, B.D., & A. Golub. 2003. Drug dependence and treatment experience among Manhattan arrestees. Presentation at American Psychological Association, Honolulu, Hawaii.

Johnson, B.D., A. Golub, & E. Dunlap. 2000. The rise and decline of drugs, drug markets, and violence in New York City, pp. 164-206. In Alfred Blumstein and Joel Wallman. (Eds.), *The Crime Drop in America.* New York: Cambridge University Press.

Johnson, P.B., S.M. Boles, H.D. Kleber, R.D. Vaughan, & K.H. McVeigh. 2000. Age-related differences in adolescent smokers and nonsmokers assessments of the relative addictiveness and health harmfulness of cigarettes, alcohol, and marijuana. *Journal of Substance Abuse.* 11(1):45-52.

Kalant, H. 2004. Adverse effects of cannabis on health: An update of the literature since 1996. *Progress in Neuro-Psychopharmacology & Biological Psychiatry.* 28(5): 849-863.

Kandel, D.B. 1973. Adolescent marijuana use: Role of parents and peers. *Science.* 181:1067-1070.

Kandel, D.B. 1974. Inter-generational and intragenerational influences on adolescent marijuana use. *Journal of Social Issues,* 30(2):107-135.

Kandel, D.B. 1980. Drug and drinking behavior among youth. *Annual Review of Sociology.* 6:235-285.

Khalsa J.H., S. Genser, H. Francis, & B. Martin. 2002. Clinical consequences of marijuana. *Journal of Clinical Pharmacology.* 42(11 Suppl):7S-10S.

Musto, D.F. 1999. *The American Disease: Origins of Narcotic Control,* 3rd ed. New York: Oxford University Press.

National Household Survey on Drug Abuse. 2003. Characteristics of new Marijuana Users. *The NHSDA Report.* SAMHSA: Substance Abuse and Mental Health Services Administration. *www.DrugAbuseStatistics.SAMHSA.gov.*

National Household Survey on Drug Abuse. 2004. Characteristics of new Marijuana Users. *The NHSDA Report.* SAMHSA: Substance Abuse and Mental Health Services Administration. *www.DrugAbuseStatistics.SAMHSA.gov.*

Parker, H. 2005. Normalization as a barometer: Recreational drug use and the consumption of leisure by younger Britons. *Addiction Research and Theory.* 13(3): 205-215.

Poulton, R., T.E. Moffitt, H. Harrington, B.J. Milne, A., & Caspi. 2001. Persistence and perceived consequences of cannabis use and dependence among young adults: Implications for policy. *New Zealand Medical Journal* 1145:544-547.

Rey, J.M., A. Martin, & P. Krabman. 2004. Is the party over? Cannabis and juvenile psychiatric disorder: The past 10 years. *Journal of the American Academy of Child and Adolescent Psychiatry.* 43(10): 1194-1205.

Schensul, J.J., C. Huebner, M. Singer, M. Snow, P. Feliciano, and L. Broomhall. 2000. The high, the money, and the fame: The emergent social context of new marijuana use among urban youth. *Medical Antropology.* 18:389-414.

Sridhar, K.S., W.A. Raub, N.L. Weatherby et al. 1994. Possible role of marijuana smoking as a carcinogen in the development of lung-cancer at a young age. *Journal of Psychoactive Drugs* 26(3): 285-288.

Substance Abuse and Mental Health Services Administration. 2003. Results from the 2002 National Survey on Drug Use and Health: National Findings. Office of Applied Studies, NHSDA Series H-22, DHHS Publication No. SMA 03-3836. Rockville, MD.

Swift, W., W. Hall, & M. Teesson. 2001. Cannabis use and dependence among Australian adults: Results from the National Survey of Mental Health and Wellbeing. *Addiction.* 96(5):737-48.

Tashkin, D.P., Baldwin, G.C., Sarafian, T., Dubinett, S., & Roth, M.D. 2002. Respiratory and immunologic consequences of marijuana smoking. *Journal of Clinical Pharmacology* 42(11 Suppl):71S-81S.

Taylor, A., and W. Hall. 2003. Respiratory health effects of cannabis: Position statement of the Thoracic Society of Australia and New Zealand. *Internal Medical Journal.* 33(7):310-3.

Wagner, F.A., & J.C. Anthony. 2002. From first drug use to drug dependence: Developmental periods of risk for dependence upon marijuana, cocaine, and alcohol. *Neuropsychopharmacology.* 26:479-488.

Zimmer, L., & Morgan, J.P. 1997. *Marijuana myths marijuana facts: A review of the scientific evidence.* New York: The Lindesmith Center

Zinberg, N.E. 1984. *Drug, Set, and Setting: The Basis for Controlled Intoxicant Use.* New Haven, CT: Yale University Press.

Zinberg, N.E., & W.M. Harding 1982. *Control Over Intoxicant Use: Pharmacological, Psychological, and Social Considerations.* New York: Human Sciences Press.

Zinberg, N.E., & J.A. Robertson. 1972. *Drugs and the Public.* New York: Simon and Schuster.

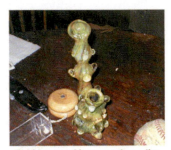

**Bubbler—smoking paraphernalia; hybrid between bong and glass pipe**

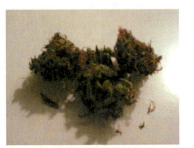

**$50 worth of Hawaiian Haze (a designer variety)**

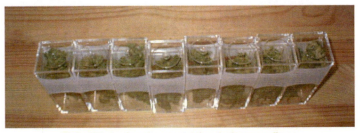

**Eight $50 plastic cubes containing designer marijuana**

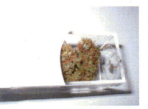

**Green indica in sealed plastic cube; retail value of $50**

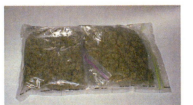

**One pound of designer marijuana (sour diesel)**

Photos taken by Flutura Bardhi

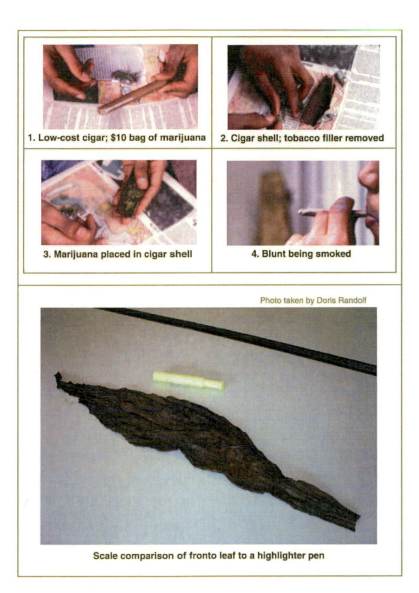

1. Low-cost cigar; $10 bag of marijuana

2. Cigar shell; tobacco filler removed

3. Marijuana placed in cigar shell

4. Blunt being smoked

Photo taken by Doris Randolf

Scale comparison of fronto leaf to a highlighter pen

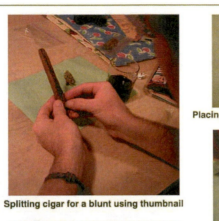

**Splitting cigar for a blunt using thumbnail**

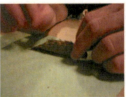

**Placing marijuana into the blunt shell**

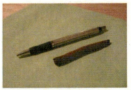

**Cigar shell filled with marijuana, ready to be rolled**

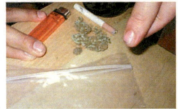

**Marijuana bud, lighter, and one hitter**

**Size comparison of a blunt to a pen**

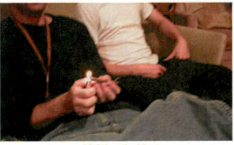

**Lighting the blunt**

Photos taken by Anthony Nguyen

# Bongs and Blunts:
# Notes from a Suburban Marijuana Subculture

Brian C. Kelly, MA, MPhil

**SUMMARY.** Bongs and blunts constitute significant elements of marijuana consumption in the United States, especially among youth. The author draws upon ethnographic methods to provide rich descriptions of these practices amongst a network of suburban marijuana users. The author first provides a description of bong use in a suburban home prior to detailing the same youth network engaging in the process of rolling and smoking a blunt in a public environment. Ultimately, the author examines and contrasts these two features of American marijuana consumption. *Article copies available for a fee from The Haworth Document Delivery Service: 1-800-HAWORTH. E-mail address: <docdelivery@haworthpress.com> Website: <http://www.HaworthPress.com> © 2005 by The Haworth Press, Inc. All rights reserved.]*

Brian C. Kelly is affiliated with Columbia University, Department of Sociomedical Sciences.

Address correspondence to: Brian C. Kelly, 722 W 168th Street, 9th Floor, New York, NY 10032 (E-mail: bck12@columbia.edu).

The author would, first and foremost, like to thank Will, Johnny, Eamon, James, Mike, and the other youth who participated in this project for allowing him into their worlds and granting him the leeway to probe various elements of their lives. He would like to thank the Department of Sociomedical Sciences for its support of this small project. He is grateful to his colleague Miguel Munoz for discussions about this project and is thankful for the comments of Jennifer Foray from her review of an earlier draft.

[Haworth co-indexing entry note]: "Bongs and Blunts: Notes from a Suburban Marijuana Subculture." Kelly, Brian C. Co-published simultaneously in *Journal of Ethnicity in Substance Abuse* (The Haworth Press, Inc.) Vol. 4, No. 3/4, 2005, pp. 81-97; and: *The Cultural/Subcultural Contexts of Marijuana Use at the Turn of the Twenty-First Century* (ed: Andrew Golub) The Haworth Press, Inc., 2005, pp. 81-97. Single or multiple copies of this article are available for a fee from The Haworth Document Delivery Service [1-800-HAWORTH, 9:00 a.m. - 5:00 p.m. (EST). E-mail address: docdelivery@haworthpress.com].

doi:10.1300/J233v04n03_04

**KEYWORDS.** Marijuana, bong, blunts, youth, white, suburbs

## INTRODUCTION

A variety of ways to consume marijuana exist. Novel methods of administration have developed over the course of the American history of marijuana use. Using a pipe to smoke marijuana and smoking marijuana in the form of a joint remain popular among Americans. Currently, youth also frequently use blunts and bongs as methods of marijuana administration, two methods that differ in certain distinctive ways. By perusing the research literature, it remains clear that the use of bongs and blunts are less well understood than other methods of administration. Despite that bong and blunt use both have become significant methods of marijuana ingestion, little published research highlights specific issues related to their use. Searches of both Medline and Psych Info reveal only 2 research-based publications related to marijuana use with the search terms for "bong" or "blunts" (Golub and Johnson, 1999; Shillington and Clapp, 2002). Thus, a significant gap exists in the research literature on these two marijuana administration methods–both key constituents of American youth consumption patterns.

The development of bongs can be traced to the Arabic Hookah, which was originally designed for smoking tobacco and still used today for that purpose. Bongs can be utilized for smoking tobacco, marijuana, and a number of other plant-based substances. Bongs function in a manner unique from other methods of marijuana administration. The bong has a basic structure. At one end is the metal bowl which contains marijuana or another substance. At the other end is the spout from which the user inhales. In between these two ends exists a cylindrical chamber in which a liquid is placed, usually water. The user inhales and draws smoke from the burning substance into the apparatus. The suction produced by inhalation draws smoke from the marijuana into the tube extending from the bowl down through the water where it is filtered. The smoke collects and hangs in the chamber. Once the user has deemed that sufficient smoke has entered the chamber, a second inhalation is made while a valve is released or a hole in the chamber uncovered. The smoke exits the chamber upward into the lungs. The filtration through water not only removes larger particulates but cools the smoke before it enters the user's mouth.

Blunts consist of marijuana rolled up in cigar paper from which the tobacco has been removed; occasionally some tobacco will be mixed in with marijuana. This method of administration derives its name from the blunt style cigars often used for this purpose, including the popular Phillies Blunts. It is estimated that blunts emerged as a form of sub-cultural style, and perhaps a reactionary one against crack use, around 1990 (Johnson, Golub, and Dunlap, 2000). Blunt use emerged in the 1980's and diffused during the 1990s through references in popular hip-hop music.[1] Though popular representations often continue to asso-ciate blunts with those involved in hip-hip youth culture, the practice of smoking blunts has expanded beyond hip-hop associated youth. NHSDA data suggest that almost half of youth who report past month usage of marijuana utilized the blunt form (Golub et al., 2004). Over the past de-cade, the market for blunts has expanded to the point where "roll your own" blunt cigar paper is now sold.

The purpose of this article is to provide a descriptive profile of the practices of bong and blunt use as methods of marijuana administration as they operate in a suburban marijuana subculture. In other words, I ex-plore how smoking bongs and blunts operates in the lives of a group of suburban youth. In the following paper, I draw upon my fieldnotes to provide rich descriptions of these marijuana practices among a group of suburban marijuana enthusiasts. The youth I describe use the drug regu-larly, in some cases almost every day, and some even deal the substance to earn cash. First, I describe an episode of bong use before I describe a blunt smoking event. The analysis that follows examines and contrasts the two practices.

Popular representations often locate drug problems within urban communities of color. Yet, marijuana usage–and most drug use for that matter–remains a pervasive issue throughout American society, includ-ing among White youth from the suburbs (Tec, 1974). Since the 1960s extensive marijuana use has been documented amongst a largely law-abiding white middle-class population (Johnson, 1973). Though per-haps contrary to popular representations, White youth may be more likely to use drugs than non-White youth. Bell et al. note that White col-lege students are significantly more likely to use marijuana than their non-White peers (1997). This evidence is further supported by NHSDA data on 12 to 17 year-olds and 18 to 25 year-olds, which shows that White youth are more likely to have used marijuana within the past month than their Black, Latino, and Asian peers (OAS, 2004). Thus, White youth remain a key population for the study of drug use. Though often captured in national surveys and college campus based research, suburban White youth remain an understudied population in the drug research literature given that the contextual facets of their lives often go without interrogation. We often bear witness to the calluses and warts in the gritty lives of the disadvantaged who use drugs; the same can hardly be said for those in more fortunate circumstances. The work from the small project described in this paper is a meek attempt to rectify this gap.

## METHODOLOGY

This study of a suburban marijuana subculture sprouted serendipitously from a study of club drug use among suburban youth.[2] I met Will, my central key informant for the marijuana subculture study, during the spring of 2003 during the course of fieldwork for a separate study on club drugs. Will used to play high school varsity basketball and he stands six feet, six inches tall. He cuts his hair close to his head, sports several tattoos, and has an air of cockiness about him. After I first met him, I arranged to interview Will about his experiences with ecstasy and other club drugs. During the course of our second interview, Will revealed the extent to which marijuana played a role in his life, both as a recreational drug and a commodity to profit from. Thereafter, I became interested in his drug dealing activities and heavy marijuana use. I gained sufficient rapport with Will and I made a trip to the North Shore of Long Island to visit his neighborhood and meet some of his "crew" [friends]. Soon, I began to conduct ethnographic fieldwork and semi-structured interviews after developing a research design and gaining IRB approval to do so. These became the two key methods by which I collected data for this study and continue to do so at present.

The hallmark of ethnographic fieldwork is the method of participant-observation. This method requires the ethnographer to spend extended periods of time participating in the lives of people in the field setting, while critically observing their habits and practices (Agar, 1980). For this project, it meant spending time with Will and his friends and meeting their families and acquaintances. Often, I was simply taken as a new friend of the crew by these family and acquaintances; Will, his friends, and I made no efforts to persuade people otherwise. The participant-observation I engaged in over an 18-month period allowed me to "hang out" with Will and his friends in the settings in which they consumed marijuana. This in-depth immersion in these settings enabled an assessment of patterns of observed behavior and the opportunity to link these observations to interview data to cultivate fuller interpretations of subcultural social norms and practices. I documented numerous occasions of their drug use. The use of participant-observation eliminated a need to rely on the self-report of these respondents; thus, it further increased the validity of the data. All fieldwork conducted during this study resulted in documentation in the form of descriptive ethnographic fieldnotes (Sanjek, 1990).

The field setting was an upper-middle class to wealthy community on the North Shore of Long Island approximately 45 minutes by commuter railroad to midtown Manhattan. The train station, which provides easy access to Manhattan as well as one of New York's two baseball stadiums, is located in the center of the community, intersecting with a main road strewn with local businesses, such as delis and restaurants. The neighborhood residents are overwhelmingly white and the heads of household are overwhelmingly professionals and business owners. Evidence of the relative wealth of the community is the seemingly endless supply of luxury cars and SUVs that dominate the local roads and driveways. Such cars are driven not merely by the heads of household in this community but by often their teenage children as well. In addition to the expensive cars, the pervasiveness of designer label clothes worn by the adults and youth alike indicates an environment of conspicuous consumption, a place where it is not simply enough to keep up with the Joneses but to outdo them as well.

In addition to my fieldwork, I augmented participant-observation with in-depth interviews. Semi-structured interviews served a dual purpose; I was able to gain retrospective data on the lives of Will and his friends, and I was able to probe their current drug practices more fully and understand the subcultural framework which guides their actions. The scope of the project as a whole and my interviewing extended beyond this network of friends, but this group and the neighborhood in which they lived comprised the key site of my fieldwork. For this reason, I draw heavily upon fieldwork amongst this network. I conducted several interviews each among Will and six of his friends. While this may appear to comprise a small "n," extensive interaction with networks of individuals over and extended period of time allows for real-time exploration and detail rich descriptions of micro-social practices (Bourgois, 1999).

The events described in the following pages occurred on separate occasions months apart. This paper is not meant to suggest that these events represent a universal manner of bong and blunt ingestion. All subcultural networks cultivate their own nuanced practices. Rather, the events in question highlight an archetypal pattern of use among these youth, comparable to other incidents in the field I have witnessed and documented.

## *BONG IN THE BASEMENT*

I hopped off the commuter rail line and called Will on his cell phone. He did not answer, so I hung out in a café near the train station for a while until I was able to reach him. Unfortunately, the café was indoors so I could not enjoy the nice June evening. He pulled up to the café where I was waiting in a brown late 80s sedan; the car of a friend of his, Eamon. Eamon, who according to Will is "half-Irish and half-Italian, but all fucked up" has short brown hair and stands at about 5' 10". He has thick shoulders like Will but seemed more chiseled; he obviously lifted weights. Eamon has a ruddy complexion and piercing eyes. We talked briefly about his having recently graduated from a small local college while Will was on the phone with a local bar placing an order for some hot Buffalo wings to bring to a friend's house (another friend, not Eamon). I realized at that point that I'd probably not get the interview done with Will that night as he seemed eager to get to his friend's place to watch the NBA draft. I wondered to myself with a sense of frustration, had I been able to get in touch with him when I first arrived in town would I have stood a better chance to interview him? I had interest in the NBA draft myself and did not want my commute to the suburbs to be for naught, so I decided to stay with them anyway.

On our short drive from the bar after picking up the Buffalo wings, Eamon and Will told me we were headed to "Mike's place." Clearly, it was the home of Mike's parents, but all of Will's friends, now adult children, act as if they own these homes. Mike is another friend of Will from the neighborhood. At the time, I presumed they knew each other growing up since their homes are only a 1/4 mile away, but couldn't say for sure. I later found out that they had only become friends in recent years.

Mike's parents had a very nice home, with a neatly manicured lawn and a new SUV parked out front. Mike lived in the furnished basement in his parent's home with access from the rear porch. After exiting the car, we walked down the driveway to the rear of the house. I made my way behind Eamon and Will. We went up into the porch in the rear of the home and then down into the basement apartment. When we arrived downstairs, we were just in time to see LeBron James selected as the first overall pick of the draft. Mike was on the couch in a robe and

James, another friend, was sitting in a lazy boy style recliner. Mike is an angry looking guy with a natural scowl on his face, standing about 5' 9" with light brown hair. He quickly changed out of his robe shortly after we arrived. Like Eamon, Mike also looked like he lifted weights. James, on the other hand, is tall and slim. He stands probably about 6' 4" and has the slim physique of a swimmer. James was much more welcoming to me than Mike was even though it was not his house. James greeted me with a smile and a handshake. He said, "Oh hey, why don't you take that seat," offering me a lounge chair positioned directly in front of the TV. "Sounds good to me," I said.

Will immediately opened up the bag of hot wings and started passing out the tins. He looked over at me and said, "You eat vegetables right?" "Yeah, why?" I replied. "Here you go. This is for you. We don't eat that trash," he said while handing me an entire tin of carrots and celery that came with the 120 hot Buffalo wings he ordered. "You sure none of you guys want any carrots and blue cheese?" I asked the rest of his crew. "Nah," they all responded while tearing into their wings. Eamon and Mike pulled a tall standing ashtray over by the couch they sat on so that they could smoke while they ate. It was one of those metal ashtrays you might find in a public facility, like an airport smoking lounge, it rose about two feet off the ground. I didn't even want to know where they took it from, so I didn't ask. After dishing out the meal, Will pulled up a chair in between where I sat and the recliner on which James was lounging about.

Eventually, when the NBA draft headed into the late 1st round, Eamon leaned over and said, "Hey Will, you got any hawks?" "Hah," Will said in a laugh, "You know I always got hawks." With that reply he went and sat on the couch by Mike and Eamon and pulled out a small bag of marijuana–roughly the size of a half-dollar. Without being asked, Mike got up and walked over by his bed. I couldn't see if he reached behind his bed or between the bed and the nightstand, but he quickly produced a large bong with "Graffix" written on it, the logo of a popular bong manufacturer. The bong was about a foot long in height and had a wide base. Extending up from the base was a long clear purplish plastic shaft; the opening at the top probably measured two inches in diameter.

Before sitting down, Mike handed the bong over to Will, who set it on the floor next to his feet. The bong just stood on the floor next to him until he was ready for it. Will seemed to be in charge. He controlled the situation with respect to the marijuana; after all, he was the supplier. As the other guys talked about basketball, Will set about pulling a few buds of marijuana out of the bag, picked at them with his fingers, and packed them into the small metal bowl at the front end of the bong. Will pushed one piece at a time down into the bowl and packed it in with his thumb; he did this with probably no more than a couple of the buds. After he completed filling the metal bowl, he eyed it for a minute, as if admiring his work. His upper lip protruded a bit as he nodded to himself in approval. He then grabbed a bottle of water off the coffee table and poured some down the plastic shaft of the bong.

Will positioned the bong between his two legs and held the tube in his left hand. James threw his lighter over to Will without being asked to do so. Will sparked the lighter in his right hand and held it over the marijuana in the small metal bowl. A warm orange glow emerged from the bowl as he inhaled deeply. A thick cloud of smoke filled the shaft of the bong. Just before taking another inhalation, Will slid the metal bowl out of a slot in front of the bong and the cloud of smoke went rushing up the purple shaft and down his throat. He held it in for a few seconds before exhaling with an exaggerated "Ahhhh." He then turned to his left and handed the bong and the lighter to Eamon.

After Eamon's inhalation, he passed the bong to Mike. The guys in succession passed the bong to their left. It made its way around the room in clockwise fashion. When each of them received the bong, he made one, and only one, large pull of smoke from the marijuana into the chamber of the bong. I noticed that James would often draw smoke into the chamber of the bong and then ingest the smoke into his lungs with several inhalations after sliding the bowl out of the base. The other guys made no issue of this but protested when Mike appeared to be initiating a second draw upon the marijuana. Mike just halted and smiled at them as if he were joking with them; it was the only time he smiled all evening.

During the bong's initial pass around the room, James held the bong up to me. I put my palm up and said, "No thanks. I appreciate it though." Will piped up, "Yeah, he can't smoke weed or anything like that because he's gonna become a doctor." "How long is it gonna be before you're a doctor?" James asked. "Probably somewhere between a year and a half and two years," I replied. "But I won't be a medical doctor though. I do health research but I'm not a medical doctor." Will cut in and said, "Yeah, he's a sociologist with anthropology. You know, sociology is all about crime and drugs and shit like that." "Oh yeah, I know. I took sociology at school," James said. Will eyed me. "You'll come and smoke weed with me after you write a book about e-pills and become a doctor?" he said, seemingly stating as matter of fact more so than asking a question. I laughed and said, "We'll have to see about that." The bong continued to make its way around the room in circular fashion, each guy taking a hit or two and then passing it along. All the while the guys smoked weed undisturbed in Mike's basement apartment, Mike's parents went about their business upstairs.

At one point, as Mike passed the bong to James on the bong's second pass around the room, the two almost managed to drop the bong. "You stupid mother fuckers," Will yelled, "What are you trying to do, ruin my night?" "Chill," James replied. "The weed is still lit." The marijuana had not become wet with bong water, which would have rendered it useless.

When the marijuana in the bong was spent, Mike held the bong and he handed back to Will. Will immediately set about to re-pack the small metal bowl with a few more buds. While Will inserted more marijuana into the bowl, Mike piped up. "Hey change the water," he said. "What do you think, I'm stupid?" Will shot back. Mike just went back to watching T.V. When the bowl was replenished, Will dumped the murky water into the garbage pail in front of the couch and refilled the chamber of the bong with fresh water. The bong then made a repeat trip around the group. They continued the circular ritual of relaying the bong to the guy to the left.

After taking hits off the bong, the guys would occasionally lean over and spit in the garbage can that had been placed in the center of the room for the purpose of collecting the bones from our Buffalo wings. There was nothing special about the guys passing around the bong. Quite frankly, they didn't even seem to be all that interested in smoking weed. Their focus primarily remained with the NBA draft. Integrating marijuana use into their other activities was just something they did as par for the course. Smoking weed was mundane for them, just another thing they did when hanging out.

Towards the end of the second bong, Will started coughing and choking on a big cloud of smoke he took in. The guys didn't even move; it was as if choking back on the smoke were just a matter of business. For the most part, they maintained a mellow atmosphere. I looked over and said, "You OK Will?" "Yeah," he replied. "I'm just a twenty-two year-old man in a 50-year-old body." That's a bit of an exaggeration but Will does seem to have his share of injuries from playing basketball as a teenager. He also seems to be a bit of a malingerer, often passing on opportunities to help out, such as when Mike's dad knocked on the door later in the evening and asked Mike to come with one friend to help move a piece of furniture. "There you go James," Will said when Mike looked back at the crew to see if he had a volunteer. James did get up to help, but I'm unsure whether this was of his own volition or because Will had already volunteered him. With that, their marijuana smoking ended for the night.

## BLUNTS IN THE BURBS

I first knew Will smoked blunts when I had seen a telltale pile of cigar tobacco on the window sill next to his bed. We stopped into his bedroom one evening so he could don a "throwback" basketball jersey before meeting up with his friends and I headed home. "So, that's part of your cigar collection huh?" I said to him as he pulled the jersey over his head. "That?" he said with a laugh, "You know what that is." Indeed, I did. The following narrative describes the process of blunt creation and usage among Will and his friend Johnny.

Will's cell phone rang. "Yeah," he muttered into his cell phone before he turned to me and said "Let's go." When we emerged from Will's mother's house, Johnny was waiting for us in his Japanese import car fitted with a racing muffler. Will and I had been watching basketball on T.V. earlier in the evening. As I climbed into the back seat, Will blurted out to Johnny, "Why are you late?" Johnny laughed. "What? Like there's something special going on tonight," he replied to Will. Then he turned to me and said, "Is this kid drunk already?" "Nah," I replied, "It's all good."

After Will lurched back into the front seat, Johnny drove off down the street. "If nothing interesting is going on, why did they convince me to go out with them tonight?" I wondered silently, realizing I should probably be in Manhattan at a club doing fieldwork for my "official" project instead of heading to a bar on Long Island with these guys. "So, what's the plan?" I asked them, hoping to get an idea of what was in store for me that evening. "What do you mean?" Johnny said. "Nothing. Never mind," I replied. "We're just going to a bar. Don't worry it's not far from the train [station]," Will interjected, perhaps sensing some of my uncertainty.

We eventually pulled into a parking lot and into one of the few remaining empty spaces. "Shit, I wish there was more light here," Johnny said. The nearest lamppost was about twenty feet away. "It'll do," Will said and pulled out a cigar from his pocket and handed it to Johnny. Johnny unwrapped the cigar from its cellophane and popped it into his mouth as he leaned back and reached into his front pocket with his right hand. He produced a small box cutter. "You always have that in your pocket?" I asked. "Yeah, why?" he replied as I remembered he works in a warehouse. I just shook my head. Will announced, "I gotta take a piss," and he hopped out of the car. Will left and walked over to a series of tall bushes lining one end of the parking lot.

While Will made use of his impromptu restroom, Johnny held the cigar lengthwise and slid the box cutter from one end to the other to open up the paper. He gently ran his thumbs along the tobacco shaft to make sure the split was complete. He then twisted his key counterclockwise in the ignition and lowered the automatic window on his side. As I sat back in the rear seat, Johnny leaned out the window with the cigar, split it open, and dumped the tobacco contents onto the ground. He wiped the remnants of tobacco off the cigar paper and sat back in the seat. Johnny raised his window and took his keys out of the ignition. By that time, Will was back in the front seat, having entered the car with an "Ahhhhhhhh, now that's more like it!"

As Will and I made idle chit chat about the basketball game, Johnny set to work licking the cigar paper. He moistened the paper so that he could roll a blunt for himself and Will. As he continued to lick the cigar paper I asked, "Doesn't that taste nasty?" "It's not too good," Johnny replied, "but it could be worse. You get used to it. Your tongue kind of gets a buzz." I still thought it was nasty.

He licked the cigar paper until it was pliable. Then Will produced a plastic bag of marijuana. He opened it and gave it a quick sniff before passing the bag over to Johnny. "Mmmm, smells tasty," he said to Johnny as he passed it over. Johnny emptied most of the bag onto the moist cigar paper sitting on his lap. He positioned the marijuana lengthwise in a long, half inch-thick strip. Johnny then asked me to grab a piece of cardboard for him from the floor of the car by the backseat. He laid the cigar paper on the piece of cardboard and used the firm surface to begin rolling the blunt. He folded the short end of the cigar paper over the marijuana and then squeezed all along the bulge of marijuana and re-folded the end of cigar paper. He repeated this process a few times. The purpose of packing it in was to get a firmly rolled blunt. When he felt it was sufficiently tight, he continued rolling it along the longer end of the cigar paper. Johnny gave it a slight twist as he finished and ran the blunt lengthwise across his moist lips. Upon completing his masterpiece, he held it up to Will for approval. Will gave him a quick nod. Johnny then held the blunt at one end, flicked his lighter, and passed it lengthwise under the blunt a few times to dry out the damp cigar paper so that they could light and smoke the blunt.

Upon completing the several passes of his lighter under the blunt, Johnny sat forward and said, "Alright, time to go for a walk." We headed towards the other end of the parking lot, which was even less well lit than where we had parked the car. On our way, we talked about the Knicks, one of our usual topics. The regular season was in its final days and Will and Johnny argued about the Knicks and their playoff chances. Johnny went into a ramble about how the Knicks were ill-equipped to go deep into the playoffs, so they were better off not going to the playoffs at all. This way, they would at least secure a better draft pick. After Johnny continued to ramble, Will interrupted him to remind him there was a more immediate task at hand. "C'mon, blaze that shit up," Will insisted as Johnny stood there with the blunt in his hand. "Oh yeah," Johnny said as he cocked his eye and the left corner of his mouth edged up in a sly grin. The grin quickly disappeared, however, as he stuck one end of the blunt in his mouth and held his lighter at the other end until it was lit. He puffed on it a few times before sticking it out in my direction. I shook my head. "You sure?" he said, as he held it up in my direction. I nodded before replying, "Don't worry, I'll let you buy me some Grey Goose (their favorite brand of vodka) when we get into the bar. I won't let your hard earned paycheck go to waste." Will stuck his hand out, wiggled his fingers towards the blunt, and declared, "The Professor has spoken! Now give me the damn blunt." Will cackled out loud, as if his comment was funnier to him than it was to the rest of us. Johnny just shook his head with a smile, then passed the blunt to Will and continued his rant. Not even seconds after the blunt left Johnny's right hand, his fingers were pulling a Marlboro out of the pack he had fished out of his pocket with his left.

As Will puffed the blunt and Johnny smoked what would be the first of two dozen cigarettes over the next couple of hours, we stood around that end of the parking lot for about ten to fifteen minutes, sometimes walking towards another spot or making ourselves look busy if a car happened to pass by. On one occasion, as an older man drove by slowly, Will cupped the blunt in his hand and lowered his arm behind his rear end as he nodded and smiled at the senior interloper. Johnny more emphatically and visually smoked his cigarette as if performing for the man in the car–which he clearly was. It was dark but they didn't want to draw any unneeded attention to themselves. They were simply getting their pre-alcohol buzz going.

Other friends waited, already drinking at a nearby bar. They expected Will and Johnny's arrival but were aware that the two probably had other things to do before heading inside. Will and Johnny passed the blunt back and forth seemingly with no rhyme or reason. Sometimes one of them held onto it for minutes at a time. When the other wanted another hit, he simply held out his hand for the blunt during the normal course of conversation. Though the centerpiece of our situation and the whole reason we were at this end of the parking lot away from the bar, Will and Johnny did not treat the blunt with any sort of significance. They merely smoked some when they wanted some.

When they were finished, some of the blunt remained. They didn't want to continue smoking the blunt and get higher than they felt they needed to be. Johnny meticulously squeezed out a red ember from the front end of the blunt and then tapped his fingers against the front end of the blunt to make sure it was extinguished. He dropped it off into the ashtray of his car before we turned around and headed into the bar. By the time I left them to catch a train back to Manhattan, they had consumed several drinks in addition to the blunt they had smoked. They smoked no more marijuana beyond the parking lot blunt as of when I left.

## *THOUGHTS ON SUBURBAN MARIJUANA PRACTICES*

These accounts describe two different marijuana practices, bong and blunt use, within the same social network. Aside from these two pervasive methods of marijuana ingestion, these youth also smoke marijuana from pipes and on rare occasions from joints. Though used for the same purpose–marijuana ingestion–certain contrasts in the practices and rationales for bong and blunt use exist. The following discussion examines the use of these methods and highlights a number of contrasting elements of bong and blunt use.

Bongs have become a staple of youth marijuana subcultures. Popular references to bong smoking arise in films and music lyrics. In most popular references as well as in practice in the lives of the youth I have shadowed, the use of bongs has a communal element to it. Youth seem to primarily engage in bong smoking when there are groups. If alone or perhaps with one other youth, they appear more likely to smoke marijuana from a pipe or perhaps a blunt.

Given that group dynamic structures the use of bongs, we witness a variety of informal rules about bong use among these youth. The immediate one is the circular nature of the bong ritual. Each youth sucks one inhalation worth of smoke into the bong chamber prior to inhalation. To take extra smoke into the chamber constitutes a violation of bong etiquette. Such violation draws rebuke from peers, as when Mike attempted to sneak a second draw of smoke and the others yelled at him. This ritual is similar to puff-puff-pass discussed among joint users in which a joint is passed in circular fashion and each recipient is permitted to puff on the joint no more than twice before passing the joint on to the next smoker. A more pragmatic instance of informal rules is the careful passing of the bong. The purpose is two-fold, so that the water does not travel up the stem to wet the marijuana and so as not to drop it. The guys allege that the water from the bong can ruin a carpet with a stain and odor.

Part of the reason that bongs remain an attractive option for marijuana consumption is that they are fairly easy to use and provide an efficient method of marijuana intake. Will noted, "I just think that some people have bongs and they keep them in their room. I guess they feel it's much easier to whip out the bong. You don't have to wait twenty minutes. You just pull the bong right out and smoke right away instead of taking the time to roll the blunt or going to the store to buy it. That's a whole long process." The use of a bong amongst a group is thus perhaps more useful for spontaneous occasions of marijuana use.

However, given certain limitations, bongs are primarily an indoor practice. Given their size, bongs usually cannot be taken elsewhere by these youth. As Will confirmed, "You know, lugging around some kind of three foot item is kind of, it gets really easy for the human eye to see." Though smaller bongs are manufactured, they nonetheless remain an inconvenient piece of drug paraphernalia that youth must carry around in order to use in other settings. Furthermore, the smell of a blunt is stronger than the use of a bong. As Will noted, "We know a couple of girls who have an apartment or a couple of guys who live with their parents but their parents could care less or the parents go away really frequent. That's about it because the smell is really harsh. You know it kind of lingers around for a couple of days." The cigar paper and unfiltered marijuana smoke make the blunt a less attractive option for those concerned about potential odor.

At the same time, smoking a bong indoors is normally not an option for these youth. Will notes, "The majority of the people, well, there's a few people whose parents could care less and let them smoke in the house, but the majority of us who live with our parents can't smoke indoors and it's much easier to smoke a blunt outside." Using a bong is a hassle unless you have sufficient privacy. As noted above, many bongs are not easily portable. They can be large and heavy. For that reason, they largely remain stashed in the bedrooms of marijuana users, unlike blunts, which are highly portable and disposable when finished.

Blunts have become a significant marijuana practice in the suburbs surrounding New York. Will asserted that a majority of his friends and acquaintances smoke blunts, which was confirmed by my observations of his friends' use. In fact, when Will was initiated into marijuana use by a junior high school classmate, he smoked marijuana in blunt form. It remains his preference. He claimed, "You know, 95% of the time I smoke [marijuana], I'll smoke a blunt." He cited White Owl, Dutchmasters, and Phillies as the most popular brands of cigars he and his friends used to roll blunts.

The use of blunts among these youth also connects to their hip-hop affiliations. A strong connection between hip-hop subcultures and blunt smoking exists (Sifaneck et al., 2003). In many respects, blunt smoking has replaced the use of joints among certain groups such as Will's crew. Will and his friends adopt blunt use much in the way that they have appropriated various other elements of hip-hop culture in their lives. However, they generally do not cop to it, since an active effort to appropriate hip-hop culture provokes claims of a lack of authenticity and assertions that one is a wannabe, their use of blunts signifies an adherence to hip-hop customs. It remains a part of hip-hop culture and corresponds to the clothing styles they wear, the music they listen to, and their linguistic repertoires.

Will also claimed a pragmatic preference for blunts. Will argues that relaxation is a primary motive for smoking marijuana. He believes that blunts are the most relaxing form of marijuana use. Blunts burn longer and do not require the continual re-ignition that a bong or a pipe would. He said, "The way I've always explained it to people and I guess they kind of agree with me. Maybe they never even thought about it and they go 'Yeah, yeah, that's right.' I think smoking is relaxing and if I was smoking out of a pipe you've got to keep re-lighting it and it gets annoying, you know. If I was on the beach for instance, I have to keep lighting it in the wind and it's almost like the point of smoking is to relax but then you're gonna be so stressed out you can't even enjoy it. So, if you smoke a blunt, you light it once and then you sit back and relax. And it has a nice little taste to it too. You can taste the weed if it's good weed. Some people prefer to smoke a bong or joints and that but I think that a blunt is always really a nice relaxing thing." Thus, the blunt is seen as more labor intensive in order to roll, but more relaxing once the process of smoking has begun.

Will also notes that if he smokes a blunt, "it has a nice little taste to it too. You can taste the weed if it's good weed." This sort of connoisseurship is important to Will and his friends since they try to purchase "hydro" and higher grade marijuana for themselves. The enjoyment of good marijuana is just as important to them as the physiological high that results. "You know, I'd rather take ten or fifteen hits and get a nice high [rather than a deep inhalation with a bong]. Sometimes with a bong you almost feel uncomfortable, it's almost like you're annihilated. I like to taste the weed too. If you smoke a bong, you only get a couple of hits. With good weed, it tastes good. You want to taste it." Will contrasts the several puffs of marijuana one might take from a blunt as opposed to the one massive "hit" you take from a bong. When inhaling from a bong, a massive dose of marijuana is delivered but not savored. He can savor good marijuana more readily with multiple puffs on a blunt. This became more vivid to me when Will pointed out that I engage in very much the same behavior when he noted that instead of gulping down shots of any old whiskey at a bar, I prefer to sip a glass of Jameson's Irish whiskey or a single-malt scotch on the rocks.

Like bong use, blunt smoking was a communal practice among these youth. Though Will and Johnny smoked a blunt just between the two of them in the parking lot behind the bar, had another friend shown up on the scene it is almost certain he would have been offered some of the blunt. Yet, the ritual element of youth passing the bong to the person on the left after no more than one inhalation differed quite considerably from the less ritualized nature of blunt smoking. Blunt smoking has less formality to it as evidenced by Will and Johnny's casual treatment of the blunt; sometimes one held onto the blunt for several inhalations rather than passing after a single inhalation. Though a shared practice, there appears to be neither a circular ritual to the practice, nor criteria for the appropriate number of inhalations. When utilized in groups larger than the incident of Will and Johnny I just described, the passing of the blunt is more active and does not sit in the hand of one user as long but the unstructured nature of blunt use remains among this network.

## NOTES

1. By the mid-1990s, references to blunt smoking could be found on hip-hop albums produced by both East Coast and West Coast artists. These albums were widely sold throughout the U.S., such as Cypress Hill's *Cypress Hill* (1991), Method Man's *Tical* (1994), and Tupac's *Me Against the World* (1995).

2. Though this project developed out of a separate study of club drug use, it was designed with the express purpose to study marijuana use and dealing in the suburbs and was subsequently monitored under a separate IRB protocol at the Columbia University Medical Center. A Certificate of Confidentiality from the National Institute on Drug Abuse was procured to further protect the confidentiality of the respondents. All names given to the respondents in this paper are pseudonyms.

# REFERENCES

Agar, M. (1980) *The Professional Stranger.* Academic Press: New York.

Bourgois, P. (1999) "Theory, Method, and Power in Drug and HIV-Prevention Research: A Participant-Observer's Critique." *Substance Use and Misuse,* Vol. 34 (14), 2153-2170.

Golub, A., and Johnson, BD. (1999) "Cohort Changes in Illegal Drug Use among Arrestees in Manhattan: From the Heroin Injection Generation to the Blunts Generation." *Substance Use and Misuse,* Vol. 34 (13), 1733-1763.

Golub, A., Johnson, B.D., Dunlap, E., and Sifaneck, S. (2004) "Projecting and Monitoring the Life Course of the Marijuana/Blunts Generation" *Journal of Drug Issues,* Vol. 34 (2), 361-388.

Johnson, B. (1973) *Marihuana Users and Drug Subcultures.* John Wiley & Sons: New York.

Johnson, B., Golub, A., and Dunlap, E. (2000) "The Rise and Decline of Hard Drugs, Drug Markets, and Violence in Inner-City New York" In Blumstein, A. and Wallman, J. (Eds.), *The Drop in Crime in America.* Cambridge Press: New York, pp. 164-206.

OAS. (2004) "Results from the 2003 National Survey on Drug Use and Health: National Findings." *DHHS Pub. # SMA 04-3964, NSDUH Series H-25.* Substance Abuse and Mental Health Services Administration: Rockville, MD.

OAS. (2002) "Results from the 2001 National Household Survey on Drug Abuse: Vol. 1, Summary of National Findings." *DHHS Pub. # SMA 02-3758.* Substance Abuse and Mental Health Services Administration: Rockville, MD.

Sanjek, R. (Ed.) (1990) *Fieldnotes: The Makings of Anthropology.* Cornell University Press, Ithaca, NY.

Shillington, A.M., and Clapp, JD. (2002) "Beer and bongs: Differential problems experienced by older adolescents using alcohol only compared to combined alcohol and marijuana use." *American Journal of Drug & Alcohol Abuse,* Vol. 28 (2), 379-397.

Sifaneck, S.J., Kaplan, C.D., Dunlap, E., and Johnson, B. (2003) "Blunts and Blowtjes: Cannabis Use in Two Cultural Settings and Their Implications for Secondary Prevention." *Free Inquiry in Creative Sociology,* Vol. 31 (1), 3-13.

Tec, N. (1974) *Grass is Green in Suburbia: A Sociological Study of Adolescent Usage of Illicit Drugs.* Libra Publishers: Roslyn Heights, NY.

# Youth Gangs and Drugs:
# The Case of Marijuana

Kathleen MacKenzie, MA
Geoffrey Hunt, PhD
Karen Joe-Laidler, PhD

**SUMMARY.** While the association between drug sales and violence has been a central focus of gang research since the 1980s, the issue of drug use within gangs has been given much less attention. This is especially true in the case of marijuana. This lack of interest is surprising given the extent to which gang members use marijuana. Other than alcohol, marijuana is the most widely used substance in gang life. In examining the culture and role of marijuana in the lives of gang members, we highlight the integration and normalization of recreational drug use within their day-to-day activities and cultural practices. In doing so, we emphasize the similarity of the role of marijuana in gangs to its role in other youth groups.

Data for this paper are drawn from the results of an on-going qualitative study of street gangs in the San Francisco Bay Area, in which 383 male gang members from three different ethnic groupings were interviewed. *Article copies available for a fee from The Haworth Document Delivery Service: 1-800-HAWORTH. E-mail address: <docdelivery@haworthpress.com> Website: <http://www.HaworthPress.com> © 2005 by The Haworth Press, Inc. All rights reserved.]*

---

Kathleen MacKenzie and Geoffrey Hunt are affiliated with the Institute for Scientific Analysis, Alameda, CA 94501.

Karen Joe-Laidler is affiliated with the University of Hong Kong, Hong Kong, SAR, China.

Address correspondence to: Geoffrey Hunt, PhD, at the above address.

[Haworth co-indexing entry note]: "Youth Gangs and Drugs: The Case of Marijuana." MacKenzie, Kathleen, Geoffrey Hunt, and Karen Joe-Laidler. Co-published simultaneously in *Journal of Ethnicity in Substance Abuse* (The Haworth Press, Inc.) Vol. 4, No. 3/4, 2005, pp. 99-134; and: *The Cultural/Subcultural Contexts of Marijuana Use at the Turn of the Twenty-First Century* (ed: Andrew Golub) The Haworth Press, Inc., 2005, pp. 99-134. Single or multiple copies of this article are available for a fee from The Haworth Document Delivery Service [1-800-HAWORTH, 9:00 a.m. - 5:00 p.m. (EST). E-mail address: docdelivery@haworthpress.com].

Available online at http://www.haworthpress.com/web/JESA
doi:10.1300/J233v04n03_05

**KEYWORDS.** Marijuana, youth gangs, ethnicity

## INTRODUCTION

Researchers and policy makers alike have defined adolescent drug use as a critical social problem. Besides its illegal nature, the reason for its importance is in part related to the belief that drug use may act as a gate-way or causal factor for future and more serious delinquency behavior. One arena within which concern about adolescent drug use has been even more heightened is that of youth gangs. While illicit drug use has been an issue with gang researchers since the 1950s (Cloward & Ohlin, 1960; Preble & Casey, 1969), it was only in the 1980s that increased attention began to focus on gang involvement in drug use. At this time as Fagan (1990) remarked: "drug use and drug dealing have been added to the stereotype of urban youth gang activities" (Fagan, 1990:183). Consequently today youth gangs are perceived as arenas within which drugs and violent behavior go hand-in-hand. As one team of gang researchers recently noted: "Drug use, drug sales and violent offending are often considered the domain of gangs and their members" (Esbensen et al., 2002:37). While many gang researchers have cautioned against any simplistic one-to-one association of violence and drug sales (Fagan, 1990; Klein & Maxson, 1989; Waldorf et al., 1993), nevertheless the pre-occupation with gangs and drug-related violence has tended to overshadow the importance of drug use itself within gangs. This may be partly due to the popular assumption that gang members use the drugs they sell (Waldorf, 1993). To date, much less research has been conducted on the social context of drug use, and especially marijuana within the social life of gangs (exceptions include Moore, 1990a, 1990b, 1991; Moore et al., 1978; Moore & Hagedorn, 1996; Padilla, 1992). This lack of interest in research on marijuana is even more surprising given the extent to which gang members use marijuana. Marijuana use, with the possible exception of alcohol, is the most widely used substance in gang life (Waldorf, 1993; Waldorf et al., 1993).

The relative neglect of a social contextual analysis of drug use stems not solely from the preoccupation with gangs and drug-related violence but is also the result of focusing on drug use from a delinquency or deviancy perspective. This approach has meant that studies of drug use within gangs, like the drug research field in general, have concentrated primarily on examining the epidemiology of drug use within gangs. While this theoretical paradigm has been important in documenting the extent of drug use within gangs, evaluating the connection between drug use and serious delinquency, and assessing the role of gangs as facilitators for increased drug use (Esbensen & Huizinga, 1993; Thornberry et al., 1993), the approach has largely ignored the culture of drug use. While not wishing to under-estimate the important contribution made by this literature to our understanding of gang life, we wish to focus in this paper on the normative aspects of gang members' lifestyles and the role and meaning of marijuana use within gangs.

Instead of examining drug use primarily as a problem behavior, we wish to analyze marijuana use as a cultural practice within the gang and consider the possible variations that exist within these cultural practices. In tracing the involvement of gang members with marijuana, we hope to highlight both the integration of recreational drug use within the day-to-day activities of gang life and the role of marijuana in the gangs. This role is similar to the role of marijuana in other youth groups, for example in leisure activities and in encouraging group solidarity (Ellickson, Collins, & Bell, 1999; Glassner, Carpenter, & Berg, 1986). In this connection, we draw from the growing body of UK studies which have shown "ordinary" young Britons perceive marijuana within a "sensible" drug taking perspective and increasingly have accommodated it into their lifestyle (Boys, Lenton, & Norcross, 1997; Measham, Parker, & Aldridge, 1998; Parker, Williams, & Aldridge, 2002). We take the view that gang members, like other young people, adopt a similar attitude toward marijuana such that its use is understood within culturally acceptable or normalized boundaries and integrated as a form of leisure and lifestyle. This paper draws from in-depth interviews from our on-going study of ethnic youth gangs in San Francisco to look at the role of marijuana within gang life. In doing so, we first trace gang members' initiation to marijuana use, and uncover the extent to which they are introduced to drugs either by family and friends outside the gang or by gang members. We then examine the integration of marijuana use into their daily lives and uncover the extent to which its use is acceptable and normalized.

## MARIJUANA USE

Marijuana is "the most widely used illicit drug in United States" according to the National Institute on Drug Abuse (NIDA, 2004). The 2001 National Household Survey on Drug Abuse (NHSDA) reports that the average age of initiation of marijuana use in 2000 was 17 years old (SAMHSA, 2002). The average age of marijuana initiates has generally declined since 1965, with the number of marijuana initiates among 12 to 17 year-olds steadily increasing from 0.8 million in 1990 to a plateau of 1.6 million per year between 1996 and 2000 (SAMHSA, 2002). In 2002, 16 percent of youth (almost 4 million) between the ages of 12 and 17 reported using marijuana in the past year (SAMHSA, 2003). Although current estimates of marijuana use are still much lower than the peak prevalence in the late 1970s, according to the Monitoring the Future study, the 1997 study also pointed to a worrying change in young people's attitudes towards marijuana. A decrease had occurred in the perceived risk of using marijuana among 12th graders although the perceived risk increased among 10th grade. This alteration had played, according to the authors, a critical role in bringing about a change in use (Johnston, O'Malley, & Bachman, 1999).

### *Marijuana and Ethnic Youth Gangs*

Although the Monitoring the Future and National Household surveys are important for providing a general overall sense of the trends in usage rates among adolescents and young adults, they have two major shortcomings in their ability to track drug use among high-risk populations, including ethnic youth gang members. First, they survey insufficient numbers of minority youth to assess adequately drug trends within these groups. This can lead to "a less than clear understanding of trends within specific minority groups over time" (Chavez et al., 1996:185). Beauvais and Oetting (2002) argue that "factors in the general adolescent culture appear to cause marijuana use rates to fluctuate over time for all American adolescents" and "factors unique to each ethnic group affect the base rates of use in that ethnic group." While drug use rates for white adolescents are generally higher than minority youth (with the exception of American Indians), the consequences of use among minorities are more severe (Wallace, 1999).

The second omission in these studies is the neglect of those students who no longer attend school. A number of different studies have reported that school drop-outs have higher rates of substance use than those students who remain in school (Annis & Watson, 1975; Elliot, Huizinga & Ageton, 1985; Fagan & Pabon, 1990; Swaim et al., 1997). As Mensch and Kandel (1988) have noted "the epidemiological data on rates of drug consumption provided annually for High School seniors in Monitoring the Future are underestimates because of the omission of school drop-outs and absentees in the data base" (1988:110). A point was confirmed by Seitz and Santos (1996), using the Youth Risk Behavior Survey, who noted that "Most national surveys do not adequately capture the risk of drug use for inner-city or disadvantaged neighborhoods" (1996:155). Consequently, these national surveys are not the best data collection methods for estimating and assessing drug use among gang members, many of whom are school drop-outs. Furthermore, as Jessor and Jessor (1977) and others (Seitz & Santos, 1996; Tec, 1974) have emphasized, drug use can be expected to be related to school drop-out since both are manifestations of "problem-proneness." Adolescents holding nonconforming attitudes and values are more likely to make the transition into deviant activities such as illicit drug use. In their study of drug use among drop-outs, Mensch and Kandel (1988) discovered that 36% of male school drop-outs and 17% of females had used marijuana more than a 100 times. These findings were also confirmed by Swaim and his associates (1997) who found that drop-outs had tried substances at rates anywhere from 1.3 to 3.0 times greater than for students who were still in school. Differences in current use was even greater. School drop-outs reported current drug use at between 1.2 to 6.4 times more than non drop-outs.

Illicit drug use has been an issue with gang researchers since the 1950s, most particularly in New York City and other urban centers when heroin and barbiturates were recognized as drugs being used by some gang members (Chein et al., 1964; Cloward & Ohlin, 1960; Feldman, 1968; Preble & Casey, 1969). However, in the 1980s, gang research increasingly focused on the sale and use of crack cocaine (Padilla, 1992; Taylor, 1989; Sanchez-Jankowski, 1991; Williams, 1989). This was largely related to the growth of crack cocaine use in the inner city and the perceived involvement of youth gangs in its distribution and sales. However, this focus has tended to overshadow, as in the general delinquency literature, the extent to which marijuana is still the most widely used illicit drug within gang life.

Gang researchers have increasingly identified drug use as the "normal pattern of street life" (Short & Strodtbeck, 1965:109), and within this culture of street life, marijuana is the most common illicit drug used (Moore, 1990b, 1991; Vigil, 1988; Waldorf, 1993). Although some researchers have described the ambivalence of some gang members and leaders towards drug use, it appears that most research shows that marijuana is both tolerated and enjoyed. As far back as the mid-1960s, Short and Strodtbeck (1965) discovered that 42.5% of African American gang members, 33.6% of white gang members used "pot." Hagedorn (1988) discovered that 60% of his sample of gang members admitted to using drugs mainly marijuana "most or all of the time, meaning at least every other day" (1988:142) and Long (1990), in his study of gang youth discovered that over 50% of his sample had used marijuana and the peak year of use was age 16. Finally, Decker and Van Winkle (1996) discovered that the use of marijuana far outweighed the use of any other illicit drug. However, while noting the extent to which gang members consumed marijuana, some researchers discovered that few differences existed in the extent of drug use between gang members and non-gang members. For instance, Fagan (1990) found that ". . . gang and non-gang youths differed little in their involvement in . . . marijuana use" (1990:202), and hence he concluded that "regular marijuana use is a natural social behavior among inner-city youths" (ibid).

### Normalization, Social Accommodation and Sensible Drug Use

The popularity of marijuana among U.S. youth and young adults in the general population as well as in high risk groups like gangs should not be surprising as it is the most widely consumed drug globally with 163 million people above the age of 15 reporting use in 2000/2001 (UNODC, 2003). In the U.K., where lifetime drug use rates are comparable to U.S. populations, researchers have observed regular and persistent use of marijuana among young people over the past decade (Parker, Williams & Aldridge, 2002). Parker, Williams and Aldridge (2002) attribute this persistent trend to the normalization of "sensible" drug use among young Britons. Their work and nearly all of the qualitative studies of youth in different regions of the U.K. have found that young people take a sensible and rational approach to drug taking whereby a cost benefits assessment is made of drug types and their differential effects and consequences (see review in Measham, Aldridge, & Parker, 2001; Parker, Williams & Aldridge, 2002). In comparison to drugs like heroin and crack cocaine, marijuana represents a drug with relatively few health, social and legal risks for "ordinary" young people (Parker, Aldridge, & Measham, 1998). This social accommodation of "sensible" recreational drug use, in particular marijuana, has been adopted by both drug users and abstainers, and has been viewed as part of a lifestyle, marked by a post-modern delay to adult status (Parker, Aldridge, & Measham, 1998; Parker, Williams, & Aldridge, 2002). The normalization of "sensible" drug use then is linked not only to the availability and access to drugs, rates of trying and using drugs, but importantly, the growing social and cultural accommodation to specific types of drugs, of which marijuana is viewed as part of the realities of postmodern life among a variety of ordinary young persons who are attached to different social groups and classes.

As mentioned above, despite the limited knowledge about the qualitative dimensions of drug use and gangs, we do know that marijuana is a prominent feature of gang life and that it is viewed in much in the same way as it is by many non-gang youth in the U.S. and the U.K. Given the fact that gangs have increasingly become a focus of research on urban youth in the United States, the task before us is to examine the social contexts of marijuana use in the gangs. This includes the processes by which gang members become initiated into marijuana use; the rationale by which gang members individually and collectively define marijuana as a sensible drug to use; the ways that it is accommodated and integrated into their leisure activities and lifestyles; and the extent to which ethnic differences exist in the roles and meanings of marijuana use.

## RESEARCH DESIGN AND SAMPLE

### Methods

The data for this article on the role of marijuana in the lives of gang members is drawn from a study on ethnic youth gangs in San Francisco between 1997 and 1999. We conducted face to face interviews with 383 self-identified male gang members who were members of 92 different gangs, of which 32 were African American, 28 were Latino, 28 Asian and Pacific Islander, and four Caucasian. Ethnicity was an important dimension of the gangs in San Francisco. Although different types of youth gangs can be found, for example, neighborhood street corner groups, drug selling groups, or formalized friendship groups, they are all organized primarily around common ethnic factors (Joe, 1993). At first glance, gangs look similar to other youth groupings in which being part of the group confers a level of affinity and commonality between individuals with similar characteristics, backgrounds and experiences. What makes gangs different is that membership carries with it a sense of identity and inherent expectations of conduct including loyalty, honor, protection and the creation and maintenance of a street reputation. A second important difference is the longevity of the groups. Gang members may spend many years in the gang, well into adulthood. As older members leave the gang, new members continue to join. Consequently, the gang has a life of its own, irrespective of changing membership.

While we discovered that some gangs had members who were of mixed ethnicity, the majority of the San Francisco gangs exhibited an ethnic characteristic. One possible explanation for this salient ethnic component was the geography of San Francisco neighborhoods, many of which had a high proportion of ethnic minority residents. The composition of gangs in each neighborhood reflected the dominant ethnic grouping of that neighborhood. Given this characteristic, our discussion will emphasize this ethnic component and where possible we will compare the different ethnicities of the gangs (see Table 1). Finally, for the purposes of this discussion we have focused on male gang members, even though young women were also members. We do this not to under-estimate the importance of the role of women in gangs but more to focus specifically on the general role of marijuana in gang life.[1]

Gang members were located using a snowball or chain referral sampling method (Biernacki & Waldorf, 1981) in which gang members referred other members of their own gangs, as well as friends and acquaintances from other San Francisco gangs, to participate in the project. In addition, our contacts with members of the community, particularly individuals who worked in schools and in community-based organizations, also referred respondents to the project enabling us to access a range of gangs in various areas in the city, albeit not necessarily representative of all ethnic youth gangs in San Francisco. Respondents were interviewed in two stages; a quantitative interview schedule followed by an in-depth focused interview. This comprehensive face to face interview covered topics ranging from basic demographic data, background and early life, family history, gang history, work and criminal histories, alcohol and drug use, drug sales to gang activities and violence. Interviews lasted, on average, two hours, and respondents received an honorarium for their participation and time. Fieldworkers conducted the interviews in a variety of settings including the respon-

TABLE 1. Social Demographic Characteristics of Homeboys by Ethnicity

| | African American (N = 177) % | Latino (N = 103) % | Asian PI (N = 79) % | Other (N = 24) % | Total (N = 383) % |
|---|---|---|---|---|---|
| *Median Age* | 19 | 18 | 18 | 19 | 18 |
| *Place of Birth* | | | | | |
| San Francisco | 84.2 | 51.4 | 36.7 | 62.5 | 64.2 |
| Other U.S City | 8.5 | 6.8 | 5.1 | 8.3 | 7.3 |
| Latin America | 0.0 | 37.9 | 0.0 | 0.0 | 10.2 |
| Hong Kong/China/Asia | 0.0 | 0.0 | 43.0 | 4.2 | 9.2 |
| Other/Unknown | 7.3 | 3.9 | 15.2 | 25.0 | 9.1 |
| *Domestic Unit before age 16* | | | | | |
| Mother and Father | 15.8 | 32.0 | 58.2 | 37.5 | 30.7 |
| Mother Only | 54.2 | 40.8 | 24.1 | 37.5 | 43.8 |
| Father Only | 5.6 | 6.8 | 3.8 | 0.0 | 5.2 |
| Mother and Stepfather | 0.6 | 1.0 | 1.3 | 0.0 | 0.8 |
| Grandparents | 15.8 | 8.7 | 0.0 | 4.2 | 9.9 |
| Other Relative | 5.1 | 1.9 | 8.9 | 12.5 | 5.2 |
| Foster Care | 1.7 | 1.0 | 0.0 | 4.2 | 1.3 |
| Other | 1.1 | 7.8 | 3.8 | 4.2 | 3.7 |
| *Education* | | | | | |
| Still in School | 36.2 | 48.5 | 38.0 | 33.3 | 39.7 |
| High School Graduate | 23.7 | 20.4 | 25.3 | 29.2 | 23.5 |
| College | 1.1 | 0.0 | 1.3 | 8.3 | 1.3 |
| Dropped Out | 39.0 | 29.1 | 34.2 | 25.0 | 34.5 |
| *Source of Income Last Month* | | | | | |
| Welfare | 1.1 | 1.9 | 2.5 | 8.3 | 2.1 |
| Job | 6.8 | 29.1 | 26.6 | 29.2 | 18.3 |
| Family | 2.2 | 15.5 | 21.5 | 8.3 | 10.2 |
| Hustle | 85.3 | 34.0 | 29.1 | 37.5 | 56.9 |
| Friends | 0.0 | 1.9 | 5.1 | 0.0 | 1.6 |
| Combination | 4.0 | 12.6 | 12.7 | 16.7 | 8.9 |
| *Marital Status* | | | | | |
| Single | 79.7 | 77.7 | 83.5 | 79.2 | 79.9 |
| Married, living with spouse | 2.2 | 4.8 | 1.2 | 4.2 | 2.9 |
| Married, not living with spouse | 2.2 | 2.9 | 0.0 | 0.0 | 1.8 |
| Living with girlfriend | 15.3 | 13.6 | 13.9 | 16.7 | 14.6 |
| *Number of Children* | | | | | |
| 0 | 71.2 | 68.0 | 94.9 | 75.0 | 75.2 |
| 1 | 17.5 | 22.3 | 1.2 | 8.3 | 15.1 |
| 2 | 7.9 | 3.9 | 1.2 | 12.5 | 5.7 |
| 3 or more | 3.4 | 5.8 | 1.2 | 4.2 | 3.7 |

dent's home, parks, coffee shops, cars, and office space in community agencies. Validity and reliability concerns were addressed in a variety of ways including rephrasing and repeating questions and cross checks on respondents' veracity through weekly staff discussions and field observations.

## Characteristics of the Sample

Almost three-quarters (274) of the respondents were born in the United States. Forty-six percent (177) of the respondents were African American, while just over a quarter (103) were Latino, and twenty-one percent were Asian/Pacific Islanders (79). The remaining twenty-four respondents were of mixed ethnicity or of other backgrounds. The age range was 13 to 50 with a median age of 18 years. Almost two-thirds of the respondents (243) were 18 or younger. The African Americans were the oldest group with a median age of 19. Asian/Pacific Islanders, Latinos and others had a median age of 18. The majority of respondents (fifty-five percent) had been involved in gangs from one to five years, a quarter from six to ten years and only five percent for less than a year (data not shown). Despite their ages, only one-fourth had completed high school. Forty-five percent of them, however, were still attending some form of educational program including GED preparation and alternative schools. The majority of the young men were single (eighty-one percent), and had no children (seventy-six percent).

The majority of the respondents were unemployed at the time of the interview, and only eighteen percent of them reported that their job was their main source of income during the last month. Overall, drug sales (hustling) represented the major source of income for fifty-seven percent of the young men. There were variations, however, among the different ethnic groups. Drug sales represented the primary income source in the last month for over eighty-five percent of the African Americans, with ninety-seven percent of African Americans admitting that they had sold drugs at some time. The median monthly income among African Americans was $1,300. By comparison, slightly more than one-third of the Latinos and approximately thirty percent of Asian Americans currently relied on drug sales for money (with more than eighty-seven percent of Latinos and more than half of Asian-Pacific Islanders having sold drugs at some time). Nearly thirty percent of Latinos and one quarter of Asian Americans relied on their job for income in the last month. These two groups reported a lower monthly median income of $600 among Latinos and $700 among Asian Americans, than did their African American counterparts, indicating that drug sales was the most lucrative income source among gang members.

Among the eighteen percent of respondents who were working either full or part-time jobs, almost half of them were in unskilled occupations. This latter characteristic reflected the occupations of the respondents' fathers, who tended to be employed in either unskilled or semi-skilled occupations, such as janitors, laborers, roofers, and cooks. Approximately twenty-seven percent of the respondents' mothers were employed, and worked in clerical, retail and service occupations, and twenty-one percent of them in either unskilled or semi-skilled occupations. Overall, our respondents were the sons of working and lower working class minority families. There were significant differences among the young men, however, in relation to their family connections and residence. Importantly, over one-half of the African American respondents reported that they lived only with their mother until at least their sixteenth birthday. Sixteen percent of them were equally as likely to live with both parents as with their grandparents. Latinos were slightly more likely to live with their mother only (forty-two percent) than with both parents (thirty-one percent). Almost sixty percent of Asian American respondents lived with both parents and one-quarter lived with only their mothers.

For the most part, the participants lived in densely populated areas of the city, areas characterized by sizeable minority and low income populations. At the time of the interview, the majority of African Americans lived in public housing. Among the other groups, however, less than one-fourth of them resided in a housing project, and instead lived in some form of private dwelling.

## STREET GANG LIFE

To understand the role of marijuana in the lives of gang members, we must begin our analysis by considering the characteristics and dynamics of street life. As many researchers have noted being on the streets is a natural and legitimized social arena for working class and minority male adolescents. For many of these young men, life is "neither the workplace nor the school; it is the street" (Messerschmidt, 1993:102). Life on the streets is governed by rules of masculinity, where notions of honor, respect and status afford outlets for expressing and defending one's masculinity. Their entree to life on the street is through the street gang. The gang epitomizes masculinity and ensures male bonding.

Once in the gang, young men gain status and respect through their ability both to assert themselves by being "street smart" and defend their fellow gang members (homeboys) by "being down." Unlike middle class boys, who can gain status and respect through academic success and participation in sports, working class minority youth gain respect through their ability to fight. Not only must they be prepared to defend themselves, and their fellow gang members, they must also be prepared to defend the reputation of their gang. Given this masculine culture of the street, what role does marijuana play?

Gang members spend the majority of their day "hanging around" (Corrigan, 1976) or "just chilling" and typically describe this activity in the very mundane terms of "doing nothing" (Hunt, Joe-Laidler, & Mac-Kenzie, 2005). Although adults perceive these activities as a waste of time, the everyday practice of "doing nothing" is, in fact, an intense and busy period of time and the activities that occur include talking, recounting details from previous events, joking, discussing business, defending one's honor, maintaining one's respect, "handling their business," fending off insults, keeping the police at bay, "cruising" around in cars, doing a few deals, defending turf, gambling and playing sports. Part of hanging out and doing nothing also involves drinking alcohol and smoking marijuana.

"Business" among gang members refers principally to drug sales. Within the social context of the gang, drug sales are viewed as a legitimate hustle and money making strategy. Hanging out in a group on the street corner provides opportunity, a place to conduct business, and a level of protection within the group. In addition to the money that drug selling can produce, drug sellers represent a lifestyle that young gang members look up to and can aspire to. The respect that sellers command, as well as the flashy clothes, cars, and girls, along with the notion that these individuals have their "stack of paper" (money) is particularly attractive to younger and less experienced male gang members in the neighborhood, who are struggling to find their place both on the street and in the local economy, where work opportunities are less appealing and less lucrative. Drug selling has been portrayed, by many gang researchers, as a way that young men both gain status and assert their masculinity–a defiant masculinity coupled with a rejection of work (Bourgois, 1996). This defiant masculinity in the form of drug dealing may lead to drug dealers being perceived as role models for young men and frequently emulated (Anderson, 1999:110), as one African American gang member illustrated.

I'm selling weed now, and it's a few weed sellers out there like Tiger, Hopper, you know what I'm saying, a few people that has been out there for ages, you know what I'm saying, you can't do nothing but respect them, like, yeah, you did that, you know what I'm saying, you one of the reasons why I'm out here right now, you know what I'm saying, I can't do nothing but respect that. (H045)

While hanging out on the streets, smoking marijuana relieves what might otherwise be a long and tedious day of standing on the corner waiting for customers. Though they generally sell their drugs as individuals rather than as a group, gang members will often "post up" together on the various street corners where sales take place, and take turns making sales. Hanging out together through the course of the day while they make their money, they pass the time rolling dice, flirting with the women passing by, and "blowin weed." Some gang members spend years in this daily routine.

"Partying" is another regular activity, where smoking marijuana has become an integral feature of gang members' leisure (Moore, 1991; Moore et al., 1978; Vigil, 1988; Vigil & Long, 1990). In fact, according to Moore (1991), "partying" for Latino gangs was synonymous with "getting high." "Getting high" for both younger and older gang members meant consuming marijuana and alcohol. Partying takes place both at public dance places in the neighborhood or at private parties held in someone's home or garage (Vigil, 1988). Private parties could be relatively spontaneous, when, for example, the group received a windfall. On these occasions, as Campbell (1990) discovered, marijuana and alcohol were purchased in bulk and the partying began. The endemic use of marijuana, especially at parties, has led some researchers, for example Moore et al. (1978), to identify it as a "party" drug, distinguishable from the use of other illicit drugs. Other internal activities include induction ceremonies where members are put through different forms of physical trials–referred to as "jumpin-in"–". . . which test member's toughness and desire for membership" (Vigil & Long, 1990:64). Initiations or "rites de passage" ceremonies are frequently accompanied by marijuana smoking (Padilla, 1992).

Within the context of street gang life, we can see the presence of marijuana throughout the daily routine, as well as its function in the underground economy among gang members. In the following sections we will explore the various arenas which contribute to the normalized use of marijuana, how marijuana is viewed and used by gang members, and how the social context of the gang furthers the normalization process.

### Starting to Use Marijuana

As Parker, Aldridge, and Measham (1998) found, availability and access to drugs are relatively easy for many young people. In our study, we found that inner city youth have access to marijuana from a variety of different sources. They can find it easily, in their schools, in their homes, in the parks, in the neighborhood and on the street corners. Given this pervasiveness, it is therefore not surprising that initiation into the use of marijuana begins at an early age for gang youth, with almost half of all respondents having tried marijuana before they became teenagers. The mean age of initiation into marijuana use was 12.4 years, with Latinos being the youngest group to have initiated marijuana use, and Asian Americans being the oldest.

More than 96 percent of all respondents had tried marijuana in their lifetime, including 98 percent of African Americans, 94 percent of Latinos, and almost 94 percent of Asian Americans. Their initiation into smoking was by and large a social activity. Few respondents had initially tried marijuana on their own, instead the vast majority had first tried it with others whether that be family members or friends.

The environment in which more than one-third of our respondents first encountered drug use was within their own family context and their own drug use was influenced by their families in a number of ways. African American respondents, more than any other ethnic group, talked about the use of drugs within their families, with more than 45 percent citing family members who used drugs. Drug use in the family households of Latinos and Asian Americans was less common than in African American homes. Slightly less than 30 percent of Latinos cited family members' drug use, and those were primarily among their siblings. Ten percent of Latinos had fathers who used, and their drug of choice was predominantly marijuana. Of the Asian American respondents, 11 percent had family members who were users (see Table 2).

Youth who grew up with drug use occurring openly within their families were curious about it even before they really understood what was involved. For these youth, marijuana was perceived as part of a normal adult social affair. As one 17 year-old African American explained:

TABLE 2. Drug Use by Ethnicity

| | TOTAL N = 383 | ASIAN/PI N = 79 | BLACK N = 177 | LATINO N = 103 | OTHER N = 24 |
|---|---|---|---|---|---|
| Mean Age First Use | NMean | NMean | NMean | NMean | NMean |
| Marijuana or hashish | 369 12.4 | 74 13.3 | 174 12.2 | 97 12.1 | 24 12.5 |
| Cigarettes | 291 13.1 | 72 12.9 | 125 13.5 | 74 12.5 | 20 13.6 |
| Glue, other inhalants | 40 13.9 | 2 13.0 | 2 11.0 | 32 14.0 | 4 14.8 |
| P.C.P., Angel dust | 45 15.1 | 4 16.8 | 2 14.5 | 31 15.1 | 8 14.5 |
| Powdered Cocaine | 137 15.4 | 21 15.5 | 36 15.9 | 64 14.9 | 16 15.9 |
| Quaaludes/Dans | 40 15.6 | 30 15.7 | N/A N/A | 2 12.5 | 8 15.9 |
| M.D.M.A or Ecstasy | 115 15.8 | 32 16.5 | 7 17.0 | 61 15.4 | 15 15.7 |
| Crank/Methamphetamine | 64 17.4 | 11 17.4 | 6 20.2 | 37 17.1 | 10 16.9 |
| L.S.D. | 81 17.6 | 25 15.7 | 8 20.9 | 29 17.7 | 9 16.1 |
| Heroin | 34 17.7 | 3 20.3 | 16 18.4 | 15 16.4 | N/A N/A |
| Crack, rock or hubba | 55 18.2 | 22 18.9 | 7 20.1 | 19 16.4 | 7 18.7 |
| Ice | 22 18.3 | 9 20.1 | 1 18.0 | 7 17.3 | 5 16.4 |
| Current Drug Use | TOTAL % | ASIAN/PI % | BLACK % | LATINO % | OTHER % |
| Marijuana or hashish | 76.8 | 65.8 | 93.8 | 59.2 | 83.3 |
| Cigarettes | 49.0 | 67.1 | 46.3 | 39.8 | 54.2 |
| P.C.P., Angel dust | 0.3 | 0.0 | 0.0 | 0.9 | 0.0 |
| Powdered Cocaine | 3.4 | 2.5 | 2.3 | 6.8 | 0.0 |
| Quaaludes/Dans | 3.4 | 11.4 | 0.0 | 0.0 | 16.7 |
| M.D.M.A or Ecstasy | 0.3 | 1.3 | 0.0 | 0.0 | 0.0 |
| Crank/Methamphetamine | 2.6 | 1.3 | 0.6 | 5.8 | 8.3 |
| L.S.D | 0.8 | 1.3 | 0.0 | 1.9 | 0.0 |
| Heroin | 2.6 | 0.0 | 3.3 | 3.9 | 0.0 |
| Crack, rock or hubba | 3.4 | 6.3 | 1.7 | 4.9 | 0.0 |
| Ice | 0.8 | 2.5 | 0.0 | 0.9 | 0.0 |

Seeing my mother, cause my father he's not really into no weed or nothing like he just drank alcohol a lot, so seeing my mother, my aunties and my uncles, just being around them. Not being around them, but you know what I'm saying, cause they didn't want us to be like, [we'd] get kicked out of the room, but for the simple fact me knowing what they was doing, I was kind of like, uh, wanting to know, curious what they was doing. You know what I'm saying? Curious of what weed would do to you, so, basically, that's how I started smoking, being around it. (H028)

In addition to growing up in a drug-using environment when they were young, five percent of the respondents gave examples of their own experiences of smoking marijuana for the first time with various family members. A 20 year-old Latino discussed his initiation into smoking at age 13 with his cousin:

> Yeah, we were up at two o'clock at night and he lighted a joint and I said, let me hit [*smoke*] that. And I kept asking him and I then I started hitting it, but I didn't know what I was doing because I didn't know how to inhale. He showed me how to inhale and what to do and then I inhaled and I started choking and I just felt my eyes close up. I don't know it felt good, I could see my toes and I started looking at my toes and it was funny because they were moving around and shit. So I was like, I like this. So I been smoking weed ever since then. (H362)

Other respondents described their first experiences with other family members, including siblings and even parents. One respondent rationalized his first experience of smoking weed with his mother by saying, "the first time I got fucked up is with my mother because she said she'd rather for me to get fucked up with her 'cuz she knows she ain't gonna get me no bullshit" (H025). Hence in some cases, the normalized use of drugs within the family household even included initiation experiences with family members, further predisposing gang members toward a view of drug use as commonplace.

The more frequent route of initiation into marijuana was through friends. It should be noted that in many circumstances friends and gang members are synonymous and it is very difficult to separate those references in text. A 16-year-old African American described how, while hanging out with neighborhood friends, he tried marijuana for the first time:

> My nigger Jimmy, my boy, the one I spent the night with when we first drank, he had some boys, and they brought some weed over, and you know, I took a drag or two, and I was sucked in. I didn't really feel affected at first, but then like a week later I wanted to try it again, and I got fucked up . . . I liked it 'cause, I don't know, it was like a different feeling that I never tried before. It was new to me. One thing I remember is after my first time of using marijuana is I had a kick out of it 'cause . . . if somebody would say somethin', I

would just crack up, and it would be just hell of funny. But nowadays I'm like immune to it. I just, I just smoke it cause it's like my second, like I don't know, like, like a second personality, it's like it's just me. I been smokin' it for so long that's what I do. (H363)

While a few of the respondents had experimented with marijuana earlier, it was during the middle school years that smoking marijuana became more common. Upon entering high school, respondents reported high levels of drug use going on at school. A young Latino was among school friends when he decided to give in and try marijuana for the first time:

The first time I smoked marijuana I was at school. I was at middle school and this one girl had a joint. She would always bring weed every day. And she would just roll it up and say, who wants to smoke weed? And everbody'd be like me, me. And she'd be smoking weed and she goes do you want to hit this? And I would be like, no I don't want that. Then fuck it, you know. I want to try it. And the first time I smoked weed I felt a little tingle the first time I smoked weed I was like oh man. And I kind of liked it. And I was like oh I like this feeling from smoking weed. (H325)

In examining initiation in to marijuana use, we find that there were a range of experiences among gang members. Some grew up in a familial context in which marijuana was socially acceptable and unproblematic and others had initiation experiences similar to non-gang youth, reported in other studies, and first tried marijuana with their peers. Whether by observing others using, hanging out with their school or neighborhood friends, or being introduced by family members, most respondents encountered marijuana in their ordinary everyday lives. Irrespective of whether they started using with family members or peers, their early initiation into using marijuana highlights the extent to which marijuana initiation may have occurred prior to joining the gang. In fact, fifty-one percent of those who had smoked weed, did so prior to hanging out with the gang. Furthermore, all other drugs were first tried when the respondents were older, indicating that once in the gang, members may have had more access and opportunity to participate in the use of other drugs. Moreover marijuana, far from being negatively stigmatized even at this stage of initiation, was for them, not stigmatized, but rather socially accepted and accommodated into the leisure activities of those around them.

## GETTING IN AND GETTING ON WITH THE GANG

Prior to describing the gang activities associated with using marijuana, let us first examine the circumstances of joining the gang. Most youth hung out with their gang prior to formally joining, some for as little as two months, and some for as long as two years. As the following table indicates, the mean age at which respondents joined the gang was slightly higher for all ethnic groups than the age at which they initiated marijuana use.

Given the fact that most San Francisco gangs are made up of adolescents and young adults who have grown up together and/or lived in the same neighborhood, it is not surprising to discover that joining the gang was a fairly informal process. Table 3 illustrates the extent to which respondents had prior exposure to gangs either as a result of school and/or neighborhood contact, or through their families. Fifty-six percent claimed that they had either grown up in the gang or had gotten in just by hanging around. "Growing up in the gang" carried with it several different connotations. By living in a neighborhood where street gang activity was commonplace, rather than atypical, involvement in the gang was a normal part of their everyday experience. Furthermore many gang members had relatives in gangs. Almost half of the respondents had immediate family members who were gang affiliated and more than two-thirds had extended family members in gangs, of which cousins, brothers and uncles were the most common.[2] Finally some groups of male youth, who had grown up and hung out together, upon reaching adolescence reframed their friendships into a more formalized association. A more formal process of joining–"jumping-in"–was more common among Latinos, three-quarters of whom were formally initiated into gangs. However, even among Latinos who were jumped in, the ascribed status of gang membership was described by one 21-year-old Latino who commented, "I was born into it . . ." (H318).

For those individuals who had not tried marijuana prior to joining a gang, once in the gang it was their fellow homeboys who would encourage them to try it, for to be in the gang and smoking marijuana was a commonplace and shared activity. For some, as in the following example, the introduction to and the use of marijuana was a natural progression from his affiliation with the gang:

> One day, my boy [homeboy] came home 'cause he used to sell drugs, and he came home and then he had some weed. And he

goes, do you wanna smoke, and I was like I ain't never smoked. And then that was it, he got me high for the first time. We smoked a whole joint. (H012)

As with other social groups, the relationship between marijuana use and getting high among gang members appears to be culturally learned (Becker, 1953). This suggests that for gang members, as is the case with other youth and social groups, socio-cultural factors are crucial in understanding this relationship and the way in which this is socially and culturally controlled and sanctioned (Becker, 1953; Feldman, Mandel, & Fields, 1985; Goode, 1970). In the process of learning to use marijuana newcomers also learn to "maintain" themselves while loaded (Glassner, Carpenter, & Berg, 1986; Schwendinger & Schwendinger, 1985).

TABLE 3. Gang Involvement by Ethnicity

| | TOTAL N = 383 | ASIAN/PI N = 79 | BLACK N = 177 | LATINO N = 103 | OTHER N = 24 |
|---|---|---|---|---|---|
| Mean Age First Joined | 14.0 | 14.7 | 13.9 | 13.5 | 14.4 |
| Joined the Gang How? | % | % | % | % | % |
| Recruited | 5.0 | 6.3 | 7.3 | 1.0 | 0.0 |
| From another group | 1.0 | 0.0 | 1.7 | 1.0 | 0.0 |
| Grew up in group | 28.5 | 21.5 | 44.1 | 7.8 | 25.0 |
| Just hung around | 28.2 | 45.6 | 30.5 | 10.7 | 29.2 |
| Jumped in | 33.2 | 17.7 | 15.3 | 74.8 | 37.5 |
| Other | 4.2 | 8.9 | 1.1 | 4.9 | 8.3 |
| Immediate Family in Gang | 48.3 | 44.3 | 42.9 | 58.3 | 62.5 |
| Extended Family in Gang | 67.9 | 62.0 | 62.7 | 78.6 | 79.2 |
| Which Family Members* | % | % | % | % | % |
| Father | 11.7 | 10.1 | 13.0 | 9.7 | 16.7 |
| Mother | 0.7 | 0.0 | 1.1 | 0.9 | 0.0 |
| Brother | 27.7 | 29.1 | 25.4 | 29.1 | 33.3 |
| Sister | 6.0 | 0.0 | 1.7 | 17.5 | 8.3 |
| Uncle | 24.3 | 26.9 | 23.2 | 23.3 | 29.2 |
| Aunt | 0.7 | 1.3 | 1.1 | 0.0 | 0.0 |
| Cousin | 46.0 | 39.2 | 41.2 | 60.2 | 41.7 |
| Other | 12.0 | 7.6 | 9.0 | 20.4 | 12.5 |

* Percentages do not add up to 100%. Some respondents cited multiple family members in gangs.

### Typical Days and Ethnic Differences

The extent to which gang members incorporated marijuana into their everyday life can be seen in their descriptions of the activities of a typical day. Seventy percent of the respondents indicated that they hung out with their homeboys daily. Even for those gang members who worked or went to school, at the end of the work day or school day they headed for the streets:

> Well, I wake up around eight. Take a shower. Get ready. Come ta school. Get outta school around 3:00. Go ta Natoma [*a street corner in the Mission district*]. Then see what I'm gonna do from there. We just smoke. Kick-it. Go home around 8:00 with some friends. Go home. Go ta sleep. And get ready for the next day. On Fridays we go out, kick-it there. Make my money. And just smoke and kick-it there. Whatever happens. . . . We sling [*sell drugs*]. We smoke. We like do sport activities. We play football sometimes and basketball. (H373)

Half of those who worked and two-thirds of those in school hung out with their homeboys on a daily basis. In fact, almost forty percent of respondents who were in school admitted to skipping out on school to get together with their gang, with school being merely a place to meet when their day began:

> Probably meet up at school or somethin like that. And then go like, you know what I'm sayin, cut . . . cut school, whatever. Go look for some weed. Go like to a little weed spot and go get some weed and like go hit the little cut [*a private area like an alley or bushes*]. Fire it up, whatever, probably, you know. (H177)

In addition to the activities of a typical day, the time spent together is important for newcomers to understand the codes of the street and the gang, and to distinguish between acceptable and unacceptable behavior. While hanging out, they learn the hierarchy of the gang and how to behave differentially with other gang members, leaders, and O.G.s (Old Gangsters). Importantly, the novitiate also learns norms around substance use within the group context.

> We got this dude, he like older than everybody, so sometimes we'll listen to what he got to say because he older than everybody.

So he knows a lot more than all the rest of the people. He'll say something like–he taught us how to roll the weed and stuff . . . . He taught us how to do a lot of stuff, go to Walgreen's or something, he was teaching us how to steal stuff; when we was like really young. (H301)

As their descriptions indicate, gang members have collectively integrated and accommodated marijuana into their everyday lifestyle. In fact, marijuana use is such an organic part of their lives that, when asked about their drug use, respondents often neglected to mention marijuana use until they were specifically probed about the substance. Gang members viewed marijuana as a substance on par with alcohol in terms of social acceptability and accessibility and many of them ". . . don't consider weed a drug, so . . . if you talkin' about weed, we always drink and smoke our weed. That's mandatory. But we don't consider that a drug" (H237).

While meeting up with the gang was the common thread in the daily lives of gang members, some differences between ethnic groups existed in both their activities and their use of drugs. Latinos reported higher use levels of cocaine, crack, methamphetamine and heroin than the other two ethnic groups, though marijuana use far outweighed any other drug. Sixty percent of Latinos were current marijuana users and one-third smoked marijuana everyday. The Latino respondents typically met up with their homeboys at their turf, whether at a park or on a street corner, early in the day. They spent the majority of their day out on the streets, sometimes hanging out in the homes of other gang members. Latinos' daily activities were generally leisurely, and on occasions, they would have picnics and BBQs in the parks, and from time to time would rent a hotel room in order to have parties. An 18-year-old recounted a typical day with the boys that with the possible exception of the drinking and marijuana smoking, seemed not that different than other adolescents:

Go to 24th street, kick back until like 3:30 everybody, all the girls will sit there until like 4, kick back, some people get high, some people get drunk, kickin' back. Try to talk to girls all day, whatever. After that, come home for a little while, kick back at home. Go back out there, chill eat, get high, then I'll call up some home boys and they'll be like, we got some girls and this and that, whatever. I'll be like, pick me up and then they'll pick me up, we'll go pick up some girls and then go kick it at a park or something, drink and get high and all that. Come back and just drop me off. That's like a normal day. Sometimes we'll go to the set [*meet with the group at their turf*] and it's hot. What we'll do, all the LNS [*the name of the gang*] girls will come out and it's hot so we'll go to Walgreens buy some water balloons, got to Tacqueria and fill up bags, and then when the girls come out we'll just start bombin' on them, we'll have a big war against the girls. That's like a hot day. We do different things all the time. (H012)

Asian American respondents were more diverse in their daily activities. They tended to sleep late and meet up with their groups in the mid-afternoon to early evenings, getting together at someone's residence or at a public place, such as a cafe, rather than out on the streets. Their daily and nightly activities also differed from African American and Latino gang members. Like the Latinos, most of their activities were leisure related, but they were more inclined toward entertainment, such as shooting pool, bowling, hanging out in coffee shops, or going to Karaoke clubs. An 18 year-old, Chinese Vietnamese gang member described a typical day with his group:

We didn't go to school. . . Like I don't know. Meet up somewhere. And go call some girls. And go to some spot like an arcade or something. Or the mall and stuff and just kick it. . . At night time . . . you know we might go to the park or something. Or somebody's house and just smoke or drink or whatever. Like sometimes we'll go to dances or something like that. Dances or clubs. (H383)

Almost two-thirds of Asian Americans were current users of marijuana, and one-third reported smoking every day. The second most commonly used drug among Asian Americans was "Dans," which referred to pharmaceutical muscle relaxants and include a variety of pills from quaaludes to percodan, currently used by more than eleven percent, followed by crack cocaine.

African American gang members were the most entrepreneurial in their daily activities. On a typical day they tended to rise early, head for the corners where they "posted up," to sell their drugs while smoking blunts (marijuana inside a cigar casing) and hanging out with their homeboys. More than eighty-five percent of the African American respondents had sold drugs in the last month, most of them on a daily basis. They often gambled together to pass the time, throwing dice being the most popular diversion. They would also occasionally go to the gym or to the courts and play basketball. While the majority of their time was spent out on the streets, they would sometimes hang out together in individuals' homes. Close to 94 percent of African Americans reported that they currently used marijuana with approximately 70 percent of African Americans reporting daily use. They were much less likely than members of either Latino or Asian American gangs to be current users of other types of drugs.

### Sensible Drug Use

African American gang members as a group were the least likely to use other drugs for several reasons. They, more than any other of the other ethnic gang members, had most clearly articulated, what Measham, Aldridge and Parker (2001) described as, a rational cost benefits assessment. African American gang members had adopted a critical and "sensible" approach to drug use because of the entrepreneurial nature of their activities around drug sales where the use of hard drugs could interfere with one's ability to make money. Marijuana was the primary drug sold by gang members with crack cocaine sales following closely behind. However, the use of crack was much lower among these gang members, who had a taboo about the use of harder drugs, "Never get high off your own supply" (H123). Sellers who also used crack soon found themselves in the hole when their use of the drug began to exceed their sales.

> Don't get strung out on them. You can sell them and hustle that is our money. When we get too involved into using them we don't make that much money and it is against the rules. Violating is going against our rules. We don't use our own drugs. (H009)

In addition, the more successful sellers didn't want to call attention to their activities and to their group by fraternizing with individuals who were obviously high and who might make trouble.

The second and perhaps even more telling reason for African Americans avoiding heavier drugs involved their having witnessed the drug use problems of family members, particularly parents. Many of these respondents whose family members had drug problems were extremely critical of those relatives, often referring to them as "fiends" or "crackheads." As one respondent suggested, "Every fiend got a family, every family got a fiend" (H116). African Americans cited the deaths of family members, incarceration, and abandonment among the deleterious effects of crack use within their families. So while marijuana use was the most prevalent among African Americans and an integral part of their daily lives as gang members on the street, other drugs, particularly crack cocaine, were viewed as disabling for individuals, for families and for the community as a whole (Boyle & Brunswick, 1980; Wallace, 1999). Most striking was the fact that more than one-fifth of African Americans had mothers who were regular drug users. Their most common drug of choice was crack cocaine, used by half of them, followed by marijuana. Among those whose mothers used crack cocaine there was a sense of abandonment and disappointment as illustrated by this 18-year-old young man, who lived in his mother's home:

> Crack, cocaine, man it's rough, no food in the house, seeing how we used to just go and have, what we would have for dinner in them days, just hoping to be some on the table for us to depend on the next day, and uh, sometimes it don't, sometimes we do, but it's like unpredictable, she unpredictable, I guess that's how she wants to be. (H151)

While some Latinos and Asian/Pacific Islanders (29% and 11% respectively) reported drug use by their family members, they did so to a significantly lesser extent than did African American respondents (48%). African Americans cited a much higher incidence of hard drug use, such as crack cocaine and heroin, among family members than did the other groups. However, some gang members identified a number of other reasons for avoiding these drugs and restricting their use to marijuana, as was expressed by an 18-year-old Latino:

> Like there's some of my homies that are older and they were crackheads. But then they left it alone. So, there's some that's can't do none. Now, it's affecting other people too. Yeah. I worry about that too. And I worry about them doing time in jail cuz of the crack, a lot a crack around. But we tell . . . I tell all homeboys that smoke crack to stop doin it. That's not right. But then some are getting into heroin now. So, that's . . . that's even worse. (H201)

Some gangs have developed rules about using drugs other than marijuana because drugs such as crack cocaine or heroin transform a person into a "dope fiend," someone who is not to be trusted and who will resort to disreputable behaviors, including potentially stealing from fellow gang members or even their own families. In some cases those individuals may be shunned by the gang because "once that friend starts using, you can't trust or rely on them to back you up" (H051). These are qualities that are counter to that of the gang member who is constantly looked upon and commands respect on the street. Marijuana use is the exception to the rule as it is perceived as a product which does not pose any harms to self, others or their business. For those gang members who were exposed through family members and some through the experiences of their gang members to the harms associated with heavier drugs like crack cocaine, marijuana has been personally and collectively understood as pleasurable, predictable, and recreational without the severe health, familial and social consequences associated with other drugs.

### *"THE BLUNTS GENERATION"*[3]

According to their own accounts, the most common method of ingesting marijuana was to smoke it in a "blunt." This consisted of emptying the tobacco from a cigar, mixing marijuana with some of the cigar tobacco and repacking the mixture into the cigar paper. One advantage to this technique was that it made the marijuana harder to detect and therefore easier to smoke while hanging out in parks, on street corners or in other public areas. This public feature of smoking blunts was aptly illustrated by a 17-year-old African American, who noted that:

> (R) If you want weed, you know what I'm sayin, you get approached on Newcomb [*a street in the neighborhood*]. Like a nigger see you walkin' down . . . he be sayin, "You need weed?" Or you could just go in the store, and there's niggers in the store that got weed for ya. . . . And then it's like we be up by the gym . . . Niggers got blunts blazin' up. Look in the car, you see a couple a females with drink. . . . And then you go in the gym, there's niggers smokin in the gym.
> (I) Now what happens when you walk in the gym . . . and they're smoking. Can you say, "Man, can you take that outside?"
> (R) Some niggers'll look at you like you crazy. It depends on how much respect you got. If you a cool nigger, they be like, "Okay, my fault. I do that for you." But if you like a nigger who ain't known . . . they'll say, "What, you crazy?" You know what I'm sayin . . . it's like that. (H051)

The increasing use of blunts has been noted by other researchers, including Golub and Johnson (1999), Johnson et al. (2000) and Schensul et al. (2000), and their increased use reflects both users' attempts to reduce the potential legal risks and community tolerance to its use. The extent of the tolerance is further illustrated by the same respondent who claimed that in certain circumstances, some police officers turned a blind eye to individuals smoking blunts, "Some of them cops is cool. They'll be like: Man, go on and smoke that" (H051).

In some African American neighborhoods where there were no stores or retail outlets, some residents purchased snacks and food items like candy, chips and sodas in bulk quantities and sold them out of their homes to their neighbors and neighborhood kids. These "candy houses" were a convenience for those individuals who didn't want to make a trip all the way to the store just to buy a candy bar. As noted by a 19 year-old African American, these entrepreneurial residents also offered consumable goods used by gang members:

> Even one of them sells beers out the candy house, beers and blunts. So say that you buy weed off the block, you ain't got to go to the store to get a blunt. It's cool, because you ain't got to walk out of your neighborhood, because when you walk out of your neighborhood is when you can get caught slipping. So you go buy a blunt, back in you all days zig zags were the thing, now it's a blunt. You cut the blunt and roll it up. So the candy houses is like the store, the neighborhood store. (H116)

One respondent even went so far as to complain about the quality of the cigars that they purchased at a local liquor store:

> We got a problem with this one store owner. They keep selling us some fucked blunts man. Giving us raggy ass blunts. You cut the blunt open and it fall apart, can't even put no weed in it. You get mad about that, that is 50 cents. You spent it for nothing. I spent 50 cents and I can't even roll it up. I get mad. They only cost 50 cents but 50 cents is a lot of money. You go spend 50 cents again that is a dollar. (H253)

As suggested in these narratives, gang members view marijuana from a "sensible" perspective, one which is associated with relatively few harms and risks when compared to other drugs available in their immediate communities. Marijuana is readily accessible, does not draw excessive attention or "heat" from the police, and appears to be somewhat tolerated in the neighborhoods and communities as evidenced by the candy house operations. Gang members have integrated marijuana into their everyday lives as a form of recreation and pleasure as well as for those special occasions of "partying." Even in comparison to alcohol, which is legally accessible and socially acceptable, some gang members perceive marijuana as a more rational choice as the latter is a pleasurable and relaxing substance which carries fewer risks of getting into confrontations with other gang members or with rival gangs. This perspective becomes even more salient for gang members when we examine some of the underlying motives for using.

## *Solidarity*

Overall, smoking marijuana was a shared group activity and an integral part of everyday life among gang members. In these everyday activities marijuana can be said to act, as in many other social groups, as a social "lubricant," or social "glue" (Becker, 1953; Fagan, 1993, 1996; Glassner, Carpenter, & Berg, 1986; Goode, 1970) working to maintain cohesion and increase solidarity within the group (Moore et al., 1978; Vigil, 1988; Vigil & Long, 1990). Marijuana also increased rapport between gang members by allowing them, while under the influence, to exhibit tender feelings for each other, feelings expressed by a 20-year-old African American:

> Oh, oh, we thick, you know what I'm saying, we thick. When I mean thick, I mean we got love for each other, like, and there's a certain respect there, like, like, . . . let me give you an example, right? Somebody who disrespecting my boys, talking about him, saying all kind of bad stuff, and I'm hearing it, right? That's my boy, I got love for him, look, I'm gonna check you about it first . . . as far as I'm concerned, you ain't gonna be sitting here talking about my boy in front of my face . . . Like that, we got love for each other like that, we down for each other like that, you look out for me, I'm gonna look out for you . . . (H045)

Latinos, more than any other group, expressed the relational aspects of their experiences in the gangs and in their drug use. They talked about using drugs for acceptance, as a means of socializing, or as one 16-year-old said, " I like to be down with them" (H209). The notion of "being down" suggests a kind of relational solidarity or camaraderie that is evident within the Latino gangs more so than in other ethnic gangs. At the same time this ethic often put pressure on individual members to engage in activities that they might otherwise have avoided. Since marijuana use is a normalized activity within the gang, some gang members felt compelled to smoke weed as a symbolic statement of belonging or as a means of establishing a street reputation. Although marijuana use was not a condition of membership, some gang members admitted that they tried drugs for the first time in order to become accepted in the group. For example, a 19-year-old African American respondent admitted, when asked why he had begun to smoke, "I was a follower, wanted to be like the other guys I was hanging with, no other reason" (H285). While this respondent was very cognizant that his motivation to smoke was tied in to a sense of belonging, others like this 18-year-old Asian American who felt pressured, had a much more complex reaction to trying drugs.

> You know, I didn't wanna do it, you know, the first time cuz, you know, cuz I didn't feel it. I didn't feel it the first time. But, you know, since there was so much peer pressure, I had–you know what I'm sayin–I had ta try it. You know what I'm saying? When I tried it, I felt, "Oh, okay, weed makes you hot, makes you feel good." (H304)

The sense of feeling bound to conform was also experienced by an 18 year-old African American when he described the pressure that gang members put on each other to join in:

> (R) If you hit it, you in. If you don't, you don't wanna be like, "No, I don't wanna hit it." The whole crew just hit it, you know, you wanna hit it too. It's pretty much the same thing with drinkin. It's pretty much a peer pressure thing . . . It's somethin that gotta be in your face. And everybody's smokin weed. You know, you could be at a party. And they're like, "Hit the joint man." You'll hit the joint. It's just . . . that's pretty much how it was.
> (I) So you never really liked it?
> (R) Nah, I never really liked it. I don't even like smokin a cigarette. Smokin is just not my thing [chuckles]. (H243)

However, the notion of peer pressure may have been an individual perception, as evidenced by, a 17-year-old Latino who described how he felt no such pressure to conform. In fact his resistance was an aspect of his street identity that gained the respect of others:

> (I) Yeah. So you're not much of a drinker or drug user though?
> (R) No.
> (I) And people respect you for that?
> (R) Yeah. That's one of the reasons–I'm different. I think that most of the people know me by . . . and I think I get more respect than other people. You know what I mean. Just because of the fact that I don't need to get drunk or to get high to be accepted. Other people do. I don't. I'm just myself. And they love me for that . . . especially the girls. (H080)

That marijuana is a shared activity within the gang, is true not only by virtue of smoking together but also in terms of obtaining drugs. Three quarters of the respondents turned to a fellow gang member, at least some of the time, when they were trying to "score" (purchase drugs), and more than one quarter bought drugs from a fellow gang member all the time. African Americans were most likely to score (85%) from a "boy" (homeboy) with 75% of Latinos and almost 70% of Asian Americans. In this regard, gang members are similar to other youth populations. As Parker, Aldridge, and Measham (1998) have shown, young people in the U.K. also relied on their networks of friends for their drug supplies. In some cases homeboys would pitch in together in order to buy weed to smoke.

> I get up, I come outside, I see my friends, they might want to "fade" on some weed. Like weed might cost five dollars, I mean ten dollars, so fade means you got to put in five and I got to put in five and then we get it. Yeah and when we do that, we probably go to my house or his house to play a game. Like Sony Playstation or something, a video game, or Nintendo 64, anyone of them just to have some fun, do something rather than just hanging out. (H117)

### Self-Medication and Escape

Gang members cited various reasons for smoking marijuana. For many, it was a sensible way to deal with the stress of being on the street and constantly having to watch one's back in case of attacks from rivals, dope fiends, potential robbers and police arrests. Most respondents believed that marijuana served to relieve stress and helped them to stay

calm, without losing focus on getting business done. Alcohol, by contrast, was not viewed as a stress relieving substance but as a chemical
pumping them up for action and bravado. "It keeps me high, it helps me
cope with the situation that's going on out here now" (H302). Marijuana
is culturally understood and defined as a relaxant, a substance to mellow
them out, and to help them to cope with real or imagined pressures.

> Really it was the stress. I was just stressed out. I was young. I had a
> kid and everything. I thought I was ready for it but I wasn't at all.
> And I don't know it was just the stress. . . Stressed out and I went to
> drugs. That was my easiest way out. You get high and do what you
> got to do and you forget about it for that time. (H135)

Asian American respondents in particular discussed the pressure they
felt from their home lives, from rules to expectations, and how drugs offered a temporary time out–the ability to disregard expectations they or
others may have, allowing them to engage fully in activities where they
do not have to think about anybody or anything. Asian Americans also indicated that they used marijuana as a disinhibitor, a means to disengage
and have fun, as a 17-year-old Laotian described:

> (R) I don't know I guess I started smoking because I wanted to be
> with them. Because I hang out with them and smoke the joints. And
> it is like I fell into . . . so I started using the drugs. Started using more
> and more. I started meeting them at T.L. in the rec centers and stuff.
> And I started hanging out. And I started seeing how, like I wanted to
> have some fun. . . We went to the park and played like tag and stuff.
> Just hang out until late at night. We was like, it was very fun. So I
> started hanging out with them more and more. And we did things to-
> gether. We started smoke . . . together. And then we started getting
> into drugs. First time smoked weed, it was scary. That is how you
> get started, you hang out and it is fun.
> (I) Your first experience smoking weed how is that? Was that?
> (R) I was so high like this, I was like in another dimension. It was
> weird, everything got slow, everything moved in slow motion. So I
> liked it. I mean I don't have to think about the problems that I have.
> Like every problem just seemed to go away. Like just relax. (H313)

Among African American respondents a common characteristic was
the notion of smoking marijuana as an escape from the realities of their
daily lives and a way of suppressing their anger at the injustices and in-
equities that they perceive when they compare their community and

their lives with the lives of others–a characteristic illustrated in the following quote:

> But, ah, hell . . . I mean, niggers ain't tryin ta stop drinkin and gettin high. You know what I'm sayin? Then what we gonna do? We gotta catch a good feelin in some way. I mean, y'all lives is good. Y'all livin fat. Y'all got good shit. Takin vacations and shit. And drivin Beamers. . . But niggers out here in the Swamp, we out here strugglin, man, and shit . . . you know, ain't nothin wrong with gettin high if you strugglin all the time. You know what I'm sayin? And feelin' bad all the time. And, you know what I'm sayin, you gotta find some kind a joy in this ol' shit. (H346)

## CONCLUSION

Within the context of street gang life in San Francisco, marijuana use is a collective activity, and has become integrated into members' everyday lives. Even before joining the gangs, smoking marijuana is, for many, a commonplace activity. Marijuana use is also present in some gang members' homes and in many family contexts, as well as in other public settings, such as schools, which suggests a cultural accommodation to marijuana. Although gang members, like those youth reported elsewhere, have accommodated marijuana into their everyday lives, the contexts of gang members' lives differ from other youth groups. The gang members in this study have had difficulties in their educational attainment and in finding legitimate and viable employment. As a result, the gang offers income-producing alternatives, primarily through drug sales which many refer to as their "job." Marijuana has been incorporated into the underground economy within the gang by being the primary drug sold by gang members, especially among African Americans, and in the idle time spent waiting for sales, marijuana is a sensible drug to use, providing relaxation, group unity, and pleasure.

While the reasons that gang members smoke marijuana vary, from self-medication, disinhibition, recreation, peer pressure and escape, being part of a gang offers the access and opportunity to do so. At the same time, such access and opportunity may also offer gang members a pathway into other drug related activities including the use of harder drugs and addiction. We have seen that even with the opportunity to use such drugs, some gangs and gang members, particularly African Americans and increasingly Latinos as well, impose social controls around the use of hard drugs, particularly in an effort to suppress the potential to interfere with the business of drug sales, as well as to maintain respect and street reputation, further illustrating the rational cost benefit assessment of drug use among gang members. One way that gang members may differ from youth described in other youth studies is that many of them have personally witnessed or experienced the devastation from drugs like crack and heroin, a factor which may also contribute to their own rationale in drug use choices.

Similar to the research about young people in the U.K., marijuana is viewed by gang members through a cost benefit assessment in which the personal health, social and legal costs are viewed as being low risks, particularly in comparison to other available drugs on the streets in their communities. Indeed, with the exception of marijuana, drug use is relatively low among most gang members, somewhat contrary to the popular portrayal of "drug crazed and drug addicted" gang members. While drugs indeed play a role in their daily lives, in terms of drug use, only marijuana was a daily patterned occurrence. Although there were individuals in each of the different ethnic groups who did participate in the use of hard drugs in addition to marijuana, for the most part gangs as a whole tried to avoid the use of heavier drugs. Gang members felt that using marijuana is not associated with unpredictability and violence, but instead, has more positive effects. It calms them down, allows them to cope with stress, and keeps them mellow. All of these characteristics point to the normalization of marijuana use within the gang context, and suggests that gang members are not so unlike other youth groups with respect to "sensible" attitudes and behaviors towards illicit drug consumption.

## NOTES

1. For a discussion of the role of young women in gangs in San Francisco see Hunt, Joe-Laidler, & Evans, 2002; Hunt, Joe-Laidler, & MacKenzie, 2000; Hunt, MacKenzie, & Joe-Laidler, 2000; Joe-Laidler & Hunt, 1997; Joe-Laidler & Hunt, 2001; and Schalet, Hunt, & Joe-Laidler, 2003.

2. For a further discussion of the relationship between family and gang see Hunt, MacKenzie, & Joe-Laidler, 2000.

3. See Golub & Johnson, 1999 and Johnson et al., 2000.

## REFERENCES

Anderson, E. (1999). *Code of the Street: Decency, Violence, and the Moral Life of the Inner City*. New York: W. W. Norton & Company.

Annis, H. M., & Watson, C. (1975). Drug use and school dropout: A longitudinal study. *Can Counselor*, 9, 155-162.

Beauvais, F., & Oetting, E. R. (2002). Variances in the etiology of the drug use among ethnic groups of adolescents. *Public Health Reports*, May-June 2002. Retrieved November 3, 2004, from http://web7.infotrac.gale/purl=rcl_ITOF_0_A95554596&dyn= 5!ar_fmt?sw_aep=montereycf.

Becker, H. S. (1953). Becoming a marijuana user. *The American Journal of Sociology*, 59, 235-242.

Biernacki, P., & Waldorf, D. (1981). Snowball sampling: Problems and techniques of chain referral sampling. *Sociological Methods and Research*, 10(2), 141-163.

Bourgois, P. (1996). *In Search of Respect: Selling Crack in El Barrio*. New York: Cambridge University Press.

Boyle, J. M., & Brunwick, A. F. (1980). What happened in Harlem? Analysis of a decline in heroin use among a generation unit of urban Black youth. *Journal of Drug Issues*, 10, 109-130.

Boys, A., Lenton, S., & Norcross, K. (1997). Polydrug use at raves by a Western Australian sample. *Drug and Alcohol Review*, 16(3), 227-234.

Campbell, A. (1990). Female participation in gangs. In C. R. Huff (Ed.), *Gangs in America* (pp. 163-182). Newbury Park, CA: Sage Publications.

Chavez, E. L., Beauvais, F., Oetting, E. R., & Deffenbacher, J. L. (1996). Drug use, violence, and victimization among White American, Mexican American, and American Indian dropouts, students with academic problems, and students in good academic standing. *Journal of Counseling Psychology*, 43, 292-299.

Chein, I., Gerard, D. L., Lee, R. S., & Rosenberg, E. (1964). *The road to heroin*. New York: Basic Books.

Cloward, R., & Ohlin, L. (1960). *Delinquency and opportunity: A theory of delinquent gangs*. New York: Free Press.

Corrigan, P. (1976). Doing nothing. In S. Hall & T. Jefferson (Eds.), *Resistance through rituals: Youth subcultures in post-war Britain* (pp. 103-105). London: Hutchinson.

Decker, S. H., & Van Winkle, B. (1996). *Life in the gang: Family, friends, and violence*. Cambridge: Cambridge University Press.

Ellickson, P. L., Collins, R. L., & Bell, R. M. (1999). Adolescent use of illicit drugs other than marijuana: How important is social bonding and for which ethnic groups? *Substance Use and Misuse*, 34(3), 317-346.

Elliott, D. S., Huizinga, D., & Ageton, S. S. (1985). *Explaining delinquency and drug abuse*. Beverley Hills: Sage Publications.

Esbensen, F.-A., & Huizinga, D. (1993). Gangs, drugs, and delinquency in a survey of urban youth. *Criminology*, 31(4), 565-589.

Esbensen, F.-A., Peterson, D., Freng, A., & Taylor, T. J. (2002). Initiation of drug use, drug sales, and violent offending among a sample of gang and nongang youth. In C. R. Huff (Ed.), *Gangs in America* (pp. 37-50). Newbury Park, CA: Sage Publications.

Fagan, J. (1990). Social processes of delinquency and drug use among urban gangs. In C. R. Huff (Ed.), *Gangs in America* (pp. 183-219). Newbury Park, CA: Sage Publications.

Fagan, J. (1993). Set and setting revisited: Influences of alcohol and illicit drugs on the social context of violent events. In S. E. Martin (Ed.), *Alcohol and interpersonal violence: Fostering multidisciplinary perspectives*, NIAAA Research Monograph 24 (pp. 161-191). Washington, DC: U.S. Government Publishing Office.

Fagan, J. (1996). Gangs, drugs, and neighborhood change. In C. R. Huff (Ed.), *Gangs in America* (pp. 39-74). Thousand Oaks and London: Sage Publications.

Fagan, J., & Pabon, E. (1990). Delinquency and school dropout. *Youth Sociology*, 20, 306-354.

Feldman, H. W. (1968). Ideological supports to becoming and remaining a heroin addict. *Journal of Health and Social Behavior*, 9, 131-139.

Feldman, H. W., Mandel, J., & Fields, A. (1985). In the neighborhood: A strategy for delivering early intervention services to young drug users in their natural environments. In A. S. Friedman & G. M. Beschner (Eds.), *Treatment services for adolescent substance abusers* (pp. 112-128). Washington, DC: U.S. Government Publishing Office.

Glassner, B., Carpenter, C., & Berg, B. (1986). Marijuana in the lives of adolescents. In G. Beschner & A. S. Friedman (Eds.), *Teen drug use* (pp. 105-123). Lexington, MA: D.C. Heath and Company.

Golub, A. L., & Johnson, B. D. (1999). Cohort changes in illegal drug use among arrestees in Manhattan: From the heroin injection generation to the blunts generation. *Substance Use and Misuse*, 34(13), 1733-1762.

Goode, E. (1970). *The marijuana smokers*. New York and London: Basic Books.

Hagedorn, J. (1988). *People and folks: Gangs, crime, and the underclass in a rustbelt city*. Chicago: Lakeview Press.

Hunt, G., Joe-Laidler, K., & Evans, K. (2002). The meaning and gendered culture of getting high: Gang girls and drug use issues. *Journal of Contemporary Drug Problems*, 29(2), 375-415.

Hunt, G., Joe-Laidler, K., & MacKenzie, K. (2000). Chillin', being dogged and getting buzzed: Alcohol in the lives of female gang members. *Drugs: Education, Prevention and Policy*, 7(4), 331-353.

Hunt, G., Joe-Laidler, K., & MacKenzie, K. (2005). Alcohol and masculinity: The case of gangs. In T. Wilson (Ed.), *Drinking culture: Alcohol and the expression of identity, class and nation* (pp. 225-254). Oxford: Berg.

Hunt, G., MacKenzie, K., & Joe-Laidler, K. (2000). I'm calling my mom: The meaning of family and kinship among homegirls. *Justice Quarterly*, 17(1), 1-31.

Jessor, R., & Jessor, S. L. (1977). *Problem behavior and psychosocial development: A longitudinal study of youth*. New York: Academy Press.

Joe, K. (1993). Issues in accessing and studying ethnic youth gangs. *The Gang Journal*, 1(2), 9-23.

Joe-Laidler, K., & Hunt, G. (1997). Violence and social organization in female gangs. *Social Justice*, 24(4), 148-169.

Joe-Laidler, K., & Hunt, G. (2001). Accomplishing femininity among the girls in the gang. *British Journal of Criminology*, 41(4), 656-678.

Johnson, B. D., Dunlap, E., Sifaneck, S. J., & Golub, A. (2000). Blunts: At the intersection of licit and illicit markets for smoking products. Working paper.

Johnston, L. D., O'Malley, P. M., & Bachman, J. G. (1999). *National survey results on drug use from the Monitoring the Future Study, 1975-1998: Volume I Secondary School Students.* Bethesda, MD: U.S. Department of Health and Human Services, National Institute on Drug Abuse.

Klein, M. W., & Maxson, C. L. (1989). Street gang violence. In M. E. Wolfgang & N. Weiner (Eds.), *Violent crime, violent criminals* (pp. 198-234). Beverly Hills: Sage Publications.

Long, J. (1990). Drug use patterns in two Los Angeles barrio gangs. In R. Glick & J. Moore (Eds.), *Drugs in Hispanic communities* (pp. 155-165). New Brunswick, NJ: Rutgers University Press.

Measham, F., Aldridge, J., & Parker, H. (2001). *Dancing on drugs.* London: Free Association Books.

Measham, F., Parker, H., & Aldridge, J. (1998). The teenage transition: From adolescent recreational drug use to the young adult dance culture in Britain in the mid-1990s. *Journal of Drug Issues, 28*(1), 9-32.

Mensch, B. S., & Kandel, D. B. (1988). Dropping out of high school and drug involvement. *Sociology of Education, 61*, 95-113.

Messerschmidt, J. W. (1993). *Masculinities and crime: Critique and reconceptualization of theory.* Lanham, MD: Rowman and Littlefield.

Moore, J. (1990a). Mexican-American women addicts: The influence of family background. In R. Glick & J. Moore (Eds.), *Drugs in Hispanic communities* (pp. 127-153). New Brunswick, NJ: Rutgers University Press.

Moore, J. (1990b). Gangs, drugs, and violence. In M. D. L. Rosa, E. Lambert, & B. Gropper (Eds.), *Drugs and violence: Causes, correlates, and consequences*, NIDA Monograph 103 (pp. 160-176). Washington, DC: U.S. Government Publishing Office.

Moore, J. (1991). *Going down to the barrio: Homeboys and homegirls in change.* Philadelphia: Temple University Press.

Moore, J., Garcia, W., Garcia, R., Cerda, C., & Valencia, L. F. (1978). *Homeboys: Gangs, drugs and prison in the barrios of Los Angeles.* Philadelphia: Temple University Press.

Moore, J., & Hagedorn, J. (1996). What happens to girls in the gang? In C. R. Huff (Ed.), *Gangs in America* (pp. 205-218). Thousand Oaks, CA: Sage Publications.

NIDA (National Institute for Drug Abuse). (2004). NIDA InfoFacts: Marijuana. Retrieved November 9, 2004, from http://www.drugabuse.gov/Infofax/marijuana.html.

Padilla, F. (1992). *The Gang as an American enterprise.* New Brunswick, NJ: Rutgers University Press.

Parker, H., Aldridge, J., & Measham, F. (1998). *Illegal leisure: The normalization of adolescent recreational drug use.* London: Routledge.

Parker, H., Williams, L., & Aldridge, J. (2002). The normalization of 'sensible' recreational drug use. *Sociology, 36*(4), 941-964.

Preble, E., & Casey, J. J. (1969). Taking care of business: The heroin user's life on the street. *The International Journal of the Addictions, 4*, 1-24.

SAMHSA (Substance Abuse and Mental Health Services Administration). (2002). *Results from the 2001 National Household Survey on Drug Abuse: Volume I. Sum-*

*mary of National Findings*. Rockville, MD: Office of Applied Studies, NHSDA Series H-17, DHHS Publication No. SMA 02-3758.

SAMHSA (Substance Abuse and Mental Health Services Administration). (2003). *Results from the 2002 National Survey on Drug Use and Health: National Findings*. Rockville, MD: Office of Applied Studies, NHSDA Series H-22, DHHS Publication No. SMA 03-3836.

Sanchez-Jankowski, M. (1991). *Islands in the street*. Berkeley: University of California Press.

Schalet, A., Hunt, G., & Joe-Laidler, K. (2003). Talking about sex with girls in the gang. *Journal of Contemporary Ethnography*, 32(1), 108-143.

Schensul, J. J., Huebner, C., Singer, M., Snow, M., Feliciano, P., & Broomhall, L. (2000). The high, the money, and the fame: The emergent social context of 'new marijuana' use among urban youth. *Medical Anthropology*, 18, 389-414.

Schwendinger, H., & Schwendinger, J. S. (1985). *Adolescent subcultures and delinquency*. New York: Praeger Special Studies.

Seitz, P., & Santos, R. (1996). Alcohol, drugs, and violence among youth, 1992. *Free Inquiry in Creative Sociology*, 24, 145-157.

Short, J. F., Jr., & Strodtbeck, F. (1965). *Group process and gang delinquency*. Chicago: University of Chicago Press.

Swaim, R. C., Beauvais, F., Chavez, E. L., & Oetting, E. R. (1997). The effect of school dropout rates on estimates of adolescent substance use among three racial/ethnic groups. *American Journal of Public Health*, 87, 51-55.

Taylor, R. C. R. (1989). The politics of prevention. In P. Brown (Ed.), *Perspectives in medical sociology* (pp. 368-389). Belmont: Wadsworth.

Tec, N. (1974). *Grass is green in suburbia: A sociological study of adolescent usage of illicit drugs*. New York: Libra.

Thornberry, T., Krohn, M., Lizotte, A., & Wierschem, D. C. (1993). The role of juvenile gangs in facilitating delinquent behavior. *Journal of Research in Crime and Delinquency*, 30, 55-87.

UNODC (United Nations Office on Drugs and Crime). (2003). *Global illicit drug trends*. New York: United Nations.

Vigil, J. D. (1988). *Barrio gangs: Street life and identity in southern California*. Austin: University of Texas Press.

Vigil, J. D., & Long, J. M. (1990). Emic and etic perspectives on gang culture: The Chicano case. In C. R. Huff (Ed.), *Gangs in America* (pp. 55-68). Newbury Park, CA: Sage Publications.

Waldorf, D. (1993). Don't be your own best customer: Drug use of San Francisco gang drug sellers. *Crime, Law and Social Change*, 19, 1-15.

Waldorf, D., Hunt, G., Joe, K., & Murphy, S. (1993). *Final report of the crack sales, gangs and violence study*. San Francisco: Institute for Scientific Analysis.

Wallace, J. M. (1999). Explaining race differences in adolescent and young adult drug use: The role of racialized social systems. *Drugs and Society*, 14(1/2), 21-36.

Williams, T. (1989). *The cocaine kids: The inside story of a teenage drug ring*. New York: Addison-Wesley Publishing.

# Social Meanings of Marijuana Use for Southeast Asian Youth

Juliet P. Lee, PhD
Sean Kirkpatrick, MA

**SUMMARY.** The paper describes findings from a pilot study of drug use and environment for Southeast Asian youths in the San Francisco Bay Area. From interviews with 31 drug-involved youths living in two low-income predominantly ethnic minority neighborhoods, smoking marijuana emerged as pervasive and highly normative. Smoking marijuana provided a means for coping with the stresses of home and community life, and located youths, moreover, within an alternative ghetto lifestyle of rap music, marijuana smoking, and youth crime, as modeled by co-resident ethnic minority peers, with which many Southeast Asian youths identified. The findings indicate the importance of the social en-

Juliet P. Lee is Research Anthropologist, Prevention Research Center, Pacific Institute for Research and Evaluation, Berkeley, CA.

Sean Kirkpatrick is Research Associate, Prevention Research Center and Program Development and Evaluation Associate, Asian Pacific Psychological Services, Richmond and Oakland, CA.

Address correspondence to: Juliet Lee, PhD, Prevention Research Center, 1995 University Avenue #450, Berkeley, CA 94704 (E-mail: jlee@prev.org).

The authors wish to thank Amy Vongthavady for assistance with recruiting and data collection, and the East Bay Southeast Asian community and service providers who supported this research.

This research was funded by grant RO3-DA15370-01 from the National Institute on Drug Abuse.

[Haworth co-indexing entry note]: "Social Meanings of Marijuana Use for Southeast Asian Youth." Lee, Juliet P., and Sean Kirkpatrick. Co-published simultaneously in *Journal of Ethnicity in Substance Abuse* (The Haworth Press, Inc.) Vol. 4, No. 3/4, 2005, pp. 135-152; and: *The Cultural/Subcultural Contexts of Marijuana Use at the Turn of the Twenty-First Century* (ed: Andrew Golub) The Haworth Press, Inc., 2005, pp. 135-152. Single or multiple copies of this article are available for a fee from The Haworth Document Delivery Service [1-800-HAWORTH, 9:00 a.m. - 5:00 p.m. (EST). E-mail address: docdelivery@haworthpress.com].

vironment as well as social status in the substance use of this group of second-generation youth. *[Article copies available for a fee from The Haworth Document Delivery Service: 1-800-HAWORTH. E-mail address: <docdelivery@ haworthpress.com> Website: <http://www.HaworthPress.com> © 2005 by The Haworth Press, Inc. All rights reserved.]*

**KEYWORDS.** Southeast Asians, drug use, adolescents, second-generation

## INTRODUCTION

A sudden drive-by, or a visit from my grandfather. Death. If some- one I know will be gone tomorrow. Will I ever wake up? . . . Noises outside. Fast-moving cars. Me or my brothers not com- ing home. What tomorrow may bring . . . [from *"Worries" by Paokeeng Saephanh*[1]]

This poem by a Laotian youth from the San Francisco Bay Area elo- quently evokes the tensions within which many second-generation Southeast Asian youth in the U.S. are growing up. From the 1970s through the 1990s, large numbers of Southeast Asians arrived in the United States as refugees; secondary migration resulted in large con- centrations of these refugees in a few states, with California having the largest numbers. Many Southeast Asian families in California have found themselves living in depressed urban or suburban areas–low-in- come and predominantly ethnic-minority neighborhoods with poor re- sources for dealing with the tremendous cultural shifts and economic challenges these immigrants have faced, but with ready availability of alcohol and other drugs and pervasive violence, crime and youth gangs. Few studies have addressed the substance use of their children. This pa- per considers the social meanings of marijuana use for these youth.

In the San Francisco Bay Area, Southeast Asian youth have been identified with poor school outcomes and other risk behaviors and are disproportionately represented in the juvenile justice system (Le, 2001; Lai, 2003; NCCD, 2003). In 2003 the death of a fifteen-year-old Lao- tian honors student in a shooting apparently targeting a drug- and gang- involved family member underlined the critical situation of Southeast Asian youth in the area.

Anthropologists from the Prevention Research Center in Berkeley conducted a pilot study of the relationships between drug use and the

social environment for Southeast Asian youths. In open-ended interviews, the researchers asked drug-involved youths to reflect on a range
of topics including their relationships with their families, peer groups,
neighborhood and school, and their knowledge of and involvement with
drugs, gangs and violence. This pilot study was intended to guide further more focused research on drug use among this population. The
findings presented here relate specifically to marijuana, the drug most
commonly reported among our respondents.

Children of new immigrants commonly feel pressured to be both
"American" and at the same time deeply and essentially of their parents'
world. For Southeast Asian youths growing up in the East Bay, the primary experience of "America" has been their neighborhoods. While the
use of marijuana is not unknown in the world of their parents, in the
world of their peers "it's everywhere," as one respondent said. Review
of our pilot data indicates that for these youths, smoking marijuana not
only provides a means of coping with the stresses of home life and the
"hard" world of their neighborhoods, but also locates youths within an
alternative "ghetto" lifestyle of rap music, marijuana smoking and
youth crime. Southeast Asian youths' use of and attitudes towards marijuana indicate that the world within which these youths are coming of
age is neither that of their immigrant parents, nor yet the U.S. mainstream, but rather the world of youth anti-heroes, the subculture of the
ghetto which is most salient in the neighborhoods within which these
youths are growing up.

## SOUTHEAST ASIANS IN THE BAY AREA

In the realm of drug research, mainland Southeast Asia has perhaps
been best known as a major site for the cultivation of the opium poppy
and the production of opiates, and there is little data on marijuana use.
Cannabis (known as *gancha* or *kancha*) has traditionally been used in
the production of textiles, and valued for its nutritional and medicinal as
well as psychoactive properties. Westermeyer listed cannabis as one of
several psychoactive substances consumed by various ethnic groups in
Laos (Westermeyer, 1988). The waterpipe commonly used in the
United States for smoking marijuana, known as a "bong," most likely
has its origins in Southeast Asia–*bong* in Thai (*bang* in Lao, *babong* in
Khmer) refers to a bamboo waterpipe used for smoking tobacco or marijuana (a practice which may traditionally be limited to older men). Others have noted the use of cannabis seeds, leaves and stalks as herbal

remedies for ailments including headache, eye strain and pain, nausea, constipation, skin disorders, and burns, and the use of hemp in ritual, particularly funerals (Clarke and Gu, 1998). Marijuana is also a common traditional ingredient in soups and curries in Indochina, and Bay Area Southeast Asians have noted that use of marijuana in cooking is not uncommon among the older generation. No studies to date have looked specifically at marijuana use among the younger generation of Southeast Asians growing up in the U.S.

"Southeast Asian" here refers to people from Laos and Cambodia as well as Vietnam, a region formerly referred to as "Indochina." Consequent to the Vietnam War, between 1975 and 1991 just over 1 million Southeast Asians had been resettled in the U.S., with the largest numbers overall settling in California.

Like other immigrants in the U.S., Southeast Asians have struggled with the many impacts of their limited English abilities, lack of education and training in applicable skills, persistent low-income status and isolation in poor and crime-ridden neighborhoods (Portes and Rumbaut, 2001). Most Southeast Asians, moreover, arrived in the U.S. having experienced multiple traumas: war, forced evacuation, forced labor, torture, lack of food or water, inadequate shelter, sexual abuse, imprisonment, stays in refugee camps of months or years, having witnessed torture, murder and executions, and separations from or deaths of family members and loved ones.[2] Many have continued to suffer from mental health problems, including depression, anxiety and post-traumatic stress disorder (Nicassio, 1985; Kroll, Habenicht et al., 1989) and have struggled with substance abuse problems that have been un- and under-diagnosed and treated, primarily abuse of alcohol, opiates and over-the-counter medications (Yee and Thu, 1987; D'Avanzo, Frye et al., 1994; Amodeo, Robb et al., 1997; D'Avanzo, 1997; O'Hare and Van Tran, 1998).

In the San Francisco Bay Area, Southeast Asians have settled in the East Bay communities of East Oakland in Alameda County and in Richmond and San Pablo in West Contra Costa County, as well as in San Francisco's Tenderloin district and the South Bay city of San Jose. These families have found themselves living in some of the poorest areas of the East Bay. Successive waves of immigrants–African Americans from the U.S. South, Mexican, and Central Americans, Southeast Asians, and more recently Eastern Europeans–have established footholds in California in declining suburban areas such as Richmond/San Pablo and East Oakland. At the 2000 census, the population of the city of Oakland was 36% African American, 31% white, 22% Latino, and

15% Asian (compared to the U.S. percentages of 12%, 75%, 13%, and 4% respectively). Twelve miles to the north along the East Bay corridor, the population of the city of Richmond in 2000 was similarly counted at 36% African American, 31% white, 27% Latino, and 12% Asian. The overall crime index (per 100,000 people) for Richmond in 2002 was 18,002, more than 4 times the national rate of 4,119, including a murder rate 13 times the national rate (77 per 100,000 people, compared to 5.6); while the overall crime index for the city of Oakland at 29,875 per 100,000 people was over 7 times the national rate, with a murder rate nearly 20 times the national rate (108 per 100,000 people) (from Federal Bureau of Investigation Crime Reports reported at www.areaconnect. com).

Southeast Asian immigrants have tried to recreate some of the social contexts of life in the old country. Many keep lush herb and vegetable gardens in tiny backyards or clusters of pots on apartment balconies; some men take weekend trips to hunt or fish. The development of ethnic enclaves through secondary migration (Miyares, 1998) has meant that populations have been large enough to support at least a minimal degree of social structure familiar from back home. Churches, temples, and senior centers have provided settings for community support groups; holidays and weddings have provided regular moments of cultural renewal for Southeast Asian adults.

Their children, however, have had to attend some of the most violent schools in some of the poorest school districts in the country. Drive-by shootings and other forms of gang violence are common; gunshots and police sirens have regularly disrupted the suburban quiet. There are few recreational and fewer employment opportunities for youths. Alcohol and drugs, on the other hand, are easily available. Drug sales have represented a viable source of income for many of the respondents of our study.

Southeast Asian refugee communities in the U.S. tend to be culturally and linguistically isolated, and somewhat insular–families and clans often attempt to address problematic issues internally. Asian families tend to see substance abuse as shameful (Kuramoto, 1995; Berganio, Tacata et al., 1997), and individuals and families are typically reluctant to seek treatment as well as to discuss their substance use issues. The pilot study was thus the research team's first approach to a population which could be considered doubly "hard to reach." In order to assess the dimensions of drug use in their neighborhoods, families and peer groups for Southeast Asian youths and peers, the investigators sought currently or formerly drug-involved youth and young adults (between the ages of 16 and 26) from Richmond/San Pablo and East Oakland as key informants. While the respondents cannot be said to represent the diversity of Southeast Asian youths in the U.S., they were remarkably thoughtful and frank, and their reflections provide useful insights into norms and attitudes related to marijuana among this understudied group.

## METHODS

Respondents were recruited through a combination of contacts with youth-serving agencies and snowball referrals. Program coordinators and counselors working with Southeast Asian youths were asked to refer youths who might fit the study criteria; after the potential respondents contacted the research team, the counselors were no longer involved and the study findings were discussed with agency staff only in the aggregate. Respondents who met the study criteria were invited to schedule an interview; upon completion of the interview, respondents were invited to refer other potential respondents. Informed consent was obtained for all respondents, and parental consent was obtained for all underage respondents. All potential respondents were screened for drug use status by self-report before being selected for an interview. All respondents were compensated for their time, and additionally received a small finder's fee for referring qualified potential respondents.

Of the 31 respondents interviewed, over a third self-identified as Cambodian, nearly a third as ethnic Mien, and approximately 20% as ethnically Lao. Respondents of mixed-ethnicity were generally mixed-Asian, e.g., one parent might be Vietnamese and the other Chinese, or Lao and Thai, etc. Nearly half the respondents were female, and over half were under age 18. Sixty-one percent of respondents came from East Oakland in Alameda County, while 32% of respondents resided in the Richmond/San Pablo area in West Contra Costa County. Eighty-one percent of respondents reported having ever used marijuana, compared to 29% who had ever used Ecstasy and 29% who had ever used other drugs (primarily methamphetamines, but cocaine and hallucinogens were also named); see Table 1. Approximately a third of the respondents had current or prior involvement with the juvenile and/or adult justice systems. Both in-school and out-of-school youths were interviewed.

The study utilized ethnographic methods to gather data on drug use and environment. In-depth confidential interviews lasting from one to two hours were conducted by two trained research assistants, both of

TABLE 1. Study respondents' background and drug use

| | N = 31 |
|---|---|
| **Ethnicity** | |
| Cambodian | 35% |
| Mien | 32% |
| Lao | 19% |
| Vietnamese | 13% |
| Mixed (non-exclusive) | 23% |
| **Age** | |
| 15-17 | 55% |
| 18-21 | 26% |
| 22-26 | 19% |
| **Gender** | |
| male | 58% |
| female | 42% |
| **Neighborhood** | |
| East Oakland | 61% |
| Richmond/San Pablo | 32% |
| other | 7% |
| **Ever Marijuana** | 81% |
| **Ever Ecstasy** | 29% |
| **Ever Other Drugs** | 29% |
| **Ever Cigarettes** | 74% |
| **Ever Alcohol** | 94% |

whom were known to Southeast Asian community members. The interviews followed a semi-structured format and covered topics including household demographics; educational experience; immigration background; sense of ethnicity; relationship with family; social networks; sense of neighborhood; availability and use of alcohol and other drugs in their neighborhoods and peer groups; experiences of gangs and violence; and sense of future. The interviewers were trained in the use of probes to deepen the quality of responses. Regular staff meetings to discuss the progress of the data collection, together with the research teams' review of incoming transcripts, allowed for emergent themes to be further explored in subsequent interviews. For example, due to concerns from the cooperating agencies that youths might be uncomfortable talking about their own drug use, respondents initially were only asked to describe drug use in their neighborhoods and peer groups in general. As it became apparent that respondents were quite comfortable and even interested in talking about their own drug use histories, such questions were included. Thus for the pilot study, drug use data for the entire sample is not available; a project collecting more detailed drug use histories and for a larger sample of Southeast Asian youth is currently underway.

All interviews were conducted in English; the interviews were tape-recorded and transcribed, and the transcripts edited by the field staff, which was particularly useful for transcribing and annotating terminology such as slang, gang name acronyms and drug names. The transcribed interviews were entered into the ATLAS.ti qualitative data management software and coded using items from the data collection instrument, as well as themes that emerged from preliminary or later analyses of the transcripts. The coded transcripts were analyzed by simple codes (e.g., "marijuana," "peer group," "drugs") and word searches (e.g., "smoke," "weed," "neighborhood") as well as meta-codes (e.g., "identity," "drug typologies," "ideology"), and by cross-referencing codes and words.

## FINDINGS

### Smoking Weed: "Everybody Does It"

Most respondents described marijuana as very prevalent in their social circles and readily available in their neighborhoods, even more so than cigarettes or alcohol: "Because weed, they don't ask you for I.D." [*Cambodian female, age 20*]. Several of our respondents themselves had sold marijuana, as well as other drugs, and many were eloquent in their knowledge of and preferences regarding available varieties of the substance.

Most of the respondents described marijuana use as a central feature of their socializing with friends ("kicking it" or "chilling"). When asked what they and their friends did when they got together, a typical response was: "Smoke weed, and take drugs. Drink. Just go to someone's house and play video games" [*mixed-ethnicity male, age 16*]. Parents and community groups in these neighborhoods have repeatedly pointed to the lack of safe and accessible public facilities or programs for youths; most respondents described hanging out at their own or friends' homes, or roaming the neighborhood:

> We used to cut school and go to one of our friend's house, and their parents not home too. So we just stay out there, hang out, drink, smoke. You know, just kick it with a lot of people, and it was fun. But then since his parents found out, we couldn't go back there no more, we end up hangin' at a cemetery, 'cause we didn't have no place to go, we just wanna be somewhere. [*Cambodian female, age 24*]

Many youths also described "hotboxing," i.e., smoking marijuana in a car with the windows rolled up, a practice prevalent in American youth culture. Respondents additionally reported smoking marijuana in "blunts," i.e., cigars or cigarillos with the tobacco filling replaced by or mixed with marijuana. The prevalence of blunt smoking in youth subcultures has been recently noted (DHHS, 1999; Golub, Johnson et al., 2004). The pilot study respondents sharply differentiated smoking marijuana, generally referred to as "weed," from use of other substances, which they called "drugs" or "dope." While smoking marijuana was described as "no big deal," use of other substances was seen as more socially stigmatized:

> You could smoke weed in front of a porch, right, and you can smell it, they wouldn't care, you know, but . . . just like, you're doin' dope, you don't want nobody to see you doin' dope. You could smoke weed, that'd be cool 'cause everybody does it, but doin' dope it's like another story. [*Cambodian female, age 24*]

Users of marijuana were similarly differentiated from users of hard drugs, referred to as "crackheads," "dopefiends," "addicts," or "narcs."[3] These attitudes are similar to reports from other studies of drug-involved youth in the U.S. and Europe (Glassner and Loughlin, 1987; Parker, Aldridge et al., 1998; Furst, Johnson et al., 1999) and may be seen as Southeast Asians youths' adoption of current and salient drug use practices and norms.

## The Ghetto Lifestyle: "You Gotta Do Hard Stuff"

Both Richmond/San Pablo and East Oakland are located in "the flats" of the East Bay Area, known for lower SES, higher levels of crime and violence, and poorer schools, compared to the more affluent communities in the East Bay hills. Many respondents reported normative violence, inter-racial tensions, and armed aggression and hostility from other residents as well as constant harassment by police in their neighborhoods. When asked to describe his neighborhood, rather than describe his physical environment, one youth described the phenomenological one:

> I mean, it's like, you always gotta look behind you. I mean, it's always like a test, you know. Life is a test, you know, they test you, you know, they look at you, they test you, they gonna come up to you, they gonna say somethin', what's up, you know, they wanna see, what's your reaction, you know just step up to the plate, and if you can't, they're gonna think you're soft, so they gonna just push you, let's see if you got any money. I mean, it's mostly people like, been in and out of jail, in and out of jail, it's like, when you get out, you have nothin'. So they try to hustle. They always try to hustle 'cause they ain't got nothin'. [*mixed-ethnicity male, age 16*]

The "code of the street" (Anderson 1998) has been described for other youths growing up in poor communities of color (Bourgois 1995; Decker and Van Winkle 1998). In social settings in which violence and aggression are constant threats, youths–particularly males but females as well–have learned to present a "macho" or "hard" self to command respect and deter aggression from others. Many respondents commented on drug preferences among youth in their neighborhoods, noting that while other youths used club drugs such as Ecstasy and psychedelics, the respondents and their peers avoided these, not only because these substances were considered "drugs," but also because they induced a subjective state of weakness which these youths could not afford. Alcohol and marijuana, on the other hand, were more associated with "hardness":

> You know how Ecstasy's like . . . I felt like I was so weak. I couldn't do nothing. I couldn't even get up and I dropped and everybody's blurry. Oh gosh, you cannot take it. . . [*Cambodian female, age 24*]

> It [Ecstasy] made you feel alright, but I felt kind of stupid, a little bit. I'm not gonna do that . . .. All my friends, they only mess with weed, that's it . . . they got all types of different weed, Light,

> Bammer, Bomb, Black Widow, Sweet Tooth . . . Mexican weed is one of the sweet kinds. All the Mexicans smoke it 'cause they like it. But if you smoke it too much, it don't hit you no more. But everyone [I know], it's like, they want to get hit hard. They smoke the other ones. You gotta do hard stuff like Black Widow, that's strong. [*mixed-ethnicity male, age 16*]

Many respondents, both male and female, identified with a ghetto youth culture, transcending ethnic lines. At the time of this study, many East Bay Southeast Asian youth dressed, carried themselves and talked in ways modeled by California African American and Latino youths. Oversized jeans and puffy down-filled jackets were standard for males and females; alternately, young women wore their jeans tight in the current style, with oversized earrings and elaborate hairstyles, and most males wore their hair buzzed short and no facial hair. Southeast Asian youths' speech patterns mirrored the dialect, rhythm and inflections of local African American youths, as did the preferred expressive art forms: rap music and poetry, particularly "gangsta" rap.

Gangsta rap emerged from the hip-hop youth subculture and music genre, but specifically featured alcohol, sex, guns, cars, and marijuana (Ross and Rose, 1994; Perkins, 1996). Gangsta rap can be seen as a salient marker of the ghetto youth culture; yet its most compelling force, at least for the respondents in the study, may have been its ability to articulate their sense of reality, the ways they experienced the world around them. When asked to whom they looked up, many respondents mentioned their parents, but others spoke of rap artists such as Tupac Shakur:

> He's like a ghetto poet. And all his raps is talking about his thug life and all that, gangster life. And it's amazing how he made a poem, it's called "A Flower That Grows in the Concrete," it's a good poem. Flower growing in the concrete, it's like, love in the ghetto, you know? And the ghetto kids running bare-feet in the street, with no shoes on, with no dirt to plant on, no trees and all that, you know, just plain street. You see a flower that grows in the concrete at a corner with a street light. That's amazing, you know? That's like, life. [*mixed-ethnicity male, age 16*]

For many youths in this study, their ghetto identity stood in sharp contrast to the world of their parents:

> They [the parents] are different 'cause, I'm like a ghetto person and they're like, you know, calm. [A ghetto person is] like, listenin' to rap music, and . . . just . . . I don't know. [*mixed-ethnicity male, age 16*]

Many youths indicated a desire to go to college, get a job to support a family; many were unsure if they would be able to attain these goals. While their parents hoped for their children to do well and help move the family out of the ghetto, the aspirations of some of their children reflected less the American dream and more the American reality as they have experienced it:

> [My future,] I don't know. I don't have one, but I have a dream though. My dream is to be a rapper, get a nice big crib, with hecka girls, hella weed . . . Yeah, one day, I'm gonna stand up on the stage and just rap for everybody, about gangsta life and all that. [*mixed-ethnicity male, age 16*]

### Stress and Drama: "Weed Makes You Forget Stuff"

When asked why, in their opinion, Southeast Asian youths used drugs and alcohol, a common response was that teens smoked marijuana because of "stress" and "drama." While drug use for stress reduction is far from unique to Southeast Asian youth, the specific contours of stress for these youths may have influenced their preference for marijuana as well as shaped the ensuing complications. "Stress and drama" included anxieties related to school, romantic relationship, friendships, as well as the stresses of the urban environment and their family situation—worries such as gunshots in the night or a visit from a grandfather cited by the young Lao poet at the opening of this paper.

Many of the study respondents indicated poor relationships with their primary families. In the East Bay, adult Southeast Asians often worked long days, perhaps holding two jobs, leaving little time or energy for their children. Language barriers existed within many families; while the first generation of immigrants had worked hard to learn English as adults, more or less successfully, most of their children spoke English as a first language and may not have been fully fluent in their parents' first language. Children often found themselves acting as *de-facto* heads of household, and performing tasks related to interacting with the outside world which would have been traditionally the domain of adults. As has been noted for other immigrant families (Portes and Rumbaut,

2001), such role reversal within families placed youth and parents in tense and often contradictory situations, with youth over-functioning for linguistically- and culturally-isolated parents. Southeast Asian youths noted that when school officials called or sent letters to inform parents of children's troubling school records, more often than not the children themselves translated–or mistranslated–these reports.

Because of this role reversal, parents may have felt they had little or no control over their children. Criminologist Tony Waters has theorized that the inability of elders to establish control over second-generation youth has historically set off waves of youthful crime in many immigrant communities in the U.S. (Waters, 1999). Older Southeast Asians have frequently complained that U.S. laws regarding child abuse prevented them from disciplining their children; role reversals and parents' depressed social statuses may have encouraged the second generation to further disregard their parents and the older generation:

> Man, we drink anywhere we want, and whatever. It don't really matter. We smoke in the house, we drink in the house, we go to other property, we drink up in the house, whatever. We do whatever we want. [*Mien male, age 16*]

Second-generation youths seeking to "fit in" with drug-using peer groups found themselves increasingly at odds with their parents. Drug use and its attendant problems–poor school performance, crime and arrest–in turn generated family drama and stress.

> One of the reasons [why kids use drugs] is that they won't fit in. The other reason is that they're really stressed 'cause they got a hard time at home or something else . . . 'Cause your parents are yelling at you for this reason and all that, then you're gonna relieve your stress, so you go to your friend's house to smoke weed, just to relax. 'Cause you know, weed makes you forget stuff. [*mixed-ethnicity male, age 16*]

Southeast Asian youths and families found themselves locked in painful cycles wherein parents' responses to the youths' lifestyles pushed youths further into use of drugs. Alienated from their families of origin, many respondents described their peer groups and particularly youth gangs as alternative families (a topic to be explored in further studies). Unfortunately, the "ghetto" lifestyle has put many youths in conflict not only with their parents' and the older generation of Southeast Asians, but with the law as well. City of Richmond police data for juveniles (age 10-17) for the year 2000 show rates of arrests for the relatively small population of Southeast Asians were strikingly similar to those for more-numerous groups in the same city: 6 arrests per 100 for Laotians, or 22 arrests for a population of 439 youths, somewhat lower than African American youths (8 in 10, or 421 arrests for 5,139 youths) but higher than for Latino youths (2 in 100, or 82 arrests for 3,477 youths) (NCCD, n.d.). While most of these arrests were for property crimes, probation officers note that most Southeast Asian youth in the system are involved with drugs, primarily marijuana.

It should be noted that many of our respondents were trying to quit their use of drugs, including marijuana, even as they upheld the ghetto ideals and represented an oppositional identity. For some, their quit attempts were due to the terms of their probation; others, however, described a consciousness change, as illustrated in the closing of a short play written by a group of Southeast Asian teens in Richmond:

> The reason I'm here is 'cause I was a young thug going around breaking the rules of the street and trying to maintain my composure. When I'm on the outs in my mind all I think of is "f– the rollers"[4] and do my thug lifestyle smoking weed and fighting with the enemy. But I noticed that everytime I do one of those crimes I end up in some place locked up. [*from "Caught Up"*[5]]

## DISCUSSION

Many studies have identified the primary role of peers and peer groups in the substance use of adolescents and young adults (Urberg, Degirmencioglu et al. 2000; Andrews, Tildesley et al. 2002; Dishion and Owen 2002; Hussong 2002). Studies of substance use and misuse among ethnic minorities, particularly immigrant populations, have additionally found acculturation to be a significant variable (Chen, Unger et al. 1999; Unger, Cruz et al. 2000). Segmented assimilation theory in particular has foregrounded the importance of the specific social milieu within which immigrants find themselves. For example, Bankston and Zhou found that Vietnamese youth growing up in inner city New Orleans tended to the patterns of risk behavior manifested by co-resident ethnic minority peers (Bankston and Zhou 1997).

The findings from our pilot study suggest that marijuana use of Southeast Asian youth may be seen in this way. Growing up in depressed suburban communities such as Richmond/San Pablo and East Oakland, they can be seen to have adopted the most salient social form around then, that of the ghetto lifestyle with its embrace of rap music and musicians, idolization of the gangsta, and normative use of marijuana as well as involvement in crime and violence.

While the literature on adolescent and young adult use of specific drugs is still somewhat underdeveloped, national datasets indicate that marijuana is one of the most commonly-used substance, along with alcohol and cigarettes (Johnston, O'Malley et al., 2003; CDC, 2004). Recent epidemiological analyses of marijuana use in U.S. urban areas have lead some scholars to propose that the 1990s represented an epidemic in marijuana use, with a vanguard of youth who tended to become involved in the justice system (Golub and Johnson, 2001). Youth who came of age in this period have consequently been referred to as the "marijuana/blunts generation" (Golub, Johnson et al., 2004). This is the era within which the children of Southeast Asian immigrants have come of age in the U.S.

Our pilot study suggests that the inclusion of Southeast Asian youth in the blunts generation reflects not only the era in U.S. history within which they came of age, and the neighborhoods within which they and their families have found themselves, but as well their own dark awareness of their social status–children of refugees and new immigrants as well as denizens of "the hood." In describing themselves as ghetto, Southeast Asian youths locate themselves not only in opposition with their parents and older generation Southeast Asians, but in opposition with the mainstream U.S. society as well. For youth unsure of their own future, from families still dealing with the repercussions of violent dislocations from their past, smoking marijuana can be a way to set aside stress as well as manifest a counter-cultural identity in a tangible and visceral way. "Chilling out" with marijuana-smoking peers can provide both a means of fitting in with other youths with similar experiences and marking oneself as "other" as well as attaining a chemically-induced respite from the worries, the stress and drama, of daily life.

As the present study is based on a small and non-random sample, the findings cannot be held to represent the marijuana use of all U.S. Southeast Asian youth. As an in-depth look at the normative role of marijuana use among these youth in urban and suburban California, the study does, however, open promising avenues for investigation. Comparisons to non-drug-using Southeast Asian peers, as well as to co-resident African American and Latino youth, from the same areas could aid in isolating the risk factors which lead to involvement with drugs. Comparisons with Southeast Asian youth in rural or small-town areas could confirm or negate the influence of the urban/suburban milieu. Finally, the pervasive role of marijuana use in the lives of these youths indicates that further attention is needed to the risky behaviors in which Asian/Pacific Islander youths may be engaging.

## NOTES

1. This poem appeared in *Quietly Torn* (Saecho, n.d., ca. 1999). The poet, a Mien teen, was a participant in the Richmond Youth Project.

2. See, for example, eloquent accounts in Faderman (1998), Szymusiak (1999) and the memoirs of Haing S. Ngor (1987), popularized in the film "The Killing Fields."

3. The respondents did not use any such label for marijuana smokers; neither, however, did the interviewers attempt to solicit such identifiers. Future studies are planned to collect data on such terminology.

4. "Rollers" are the police in street slang (www.blackstate.com/allthingsghetto/ghettoslangdic).

5. The script for this play, written by a collective of Mien teens participating in the Richmond Youth Project, appeared in *Quietly Torn* (Saecho n.d., ca. 1999).

## REFERENCES

Amodeo, M., & N. Robb et al. (1997). "Alcohol and other drug problems among Southeast Asians: Patterns of use and approaches to assessment and intervention." *Alcoholism Treatment Quarterly* 15(3).

Anderson, E. (1998). "The social ecology of youth violence." *Youth Violence.* M. H. Tonry and M. H. Moore. Chicago, IL, University of Chicago Press. 24: 65-104.

Andrews, J. A., & E. Tildesley et al. (2002). "Influence of peers on young adult substance use." *Health Psychology* 21(4): 349-357.

Bankston, C. L. and M. Zhou (1997). "The social adjustment of Vietnamese American adolescents: Evidence for a segmented assimilation approach." *Social Science Quarterly* 78(2): 508-523.

Berganio, J. T. J., L. A. Tacata, Jr. et al. (1997). "The prevalence and impact of alcohol, tobacco, and other drugs on Filipino American communities." *Filipino Americans: Transformation and Identity.* E. Maria, P. P. Root and et al. Thousand Oaks, CA: USA: 272-286.

Bourgois, P. (1995). *In Search of Respect: Selling Crack in El Barrio.* Cambridge, UK: Cambridge University Press.

CDC (2004). Youth Risk Behavior Surveillance–United States, 2003, Centers for Disease Control and Prevention.

Chen, X., J. B. Unger et al. (1999). "Smoking patterns of Asian-American youth in California and their relationship with acculturation." *Journal of Adolescent Health* 24(5): 321-328.

Clarke, R. C., and W. Gu (1998). "Survey of hemp (Cannabis sativa l.) use by the Hmong (Miao) of the China/Vietnam border region." *Journal of the International Hemp Association* 5(1): 4-9.

D'Avanzo, C. E. (1997). "Southeast Asians: Asian-Pacific Americans at risk for substance misuse." *Substance Use Misuse* 32(7-8): 829-48.

D'Avanzo, C. E., B. Frye et al. (1994). "Culture, stress, and substance use in Cambodian refugee women." *Journal of Studies on Alcohol* 55(4): 420-6.

Decker, S. H., and B. Van Winkle (1998). *Life in the Gang: Family, Friends, and Violence.* Cambridge, UK: Cambridge University Press.

DHHS (1999). Youth use of cigars: Patterns of use and perceptions of risk. Bethesda MD: Department of Health and Human Services, Office of Inspector General.

Dishion, T. J., and L. D. Owen (2002). "Longitudinal analysis of friendships and substance use: Bidirectional influence from adolescence to adulthood." *Developmental Psychology* 38(4): 480-491.

Faderman, L., and G. Xiong (Eds.) (1998). *I Begin My Life All Over Again: The Hmong and the American Immigrant Experience.* Boston: Beacon Press.

Furst, R. T., B. D. Johnson et al. (1999). The stigmatized image of the "crack head": A sociocultural exploration of a barrier to cocaine smoking among a cohort of youth in New York City. *Deviant Behavior* 20: 153-181.

Glassner, B., and J. Loughlin (1987). *Drug Use in Adolescent Worlds: Burnouts to Straights.* New York: St. Martin's Press, Inc.

Golub, A., and B. D. Johnson (2001). The rise of marijuana as the drug of choice among youthful adult arrestees. Washington, DC: National Institute of Justice.

Golub, A., B. D. Johnson et al. (2004). "Projecting the life course of the marijuana/blunts generation." *Journal of Drug Issues* 4(2): 361-388.

Hussong, A. M. (2002). "Differentiating peer contexts and risk for adolescent substance use." *Journal of Youth & Adolescence* 31(3): 207-220.

Johnston, L. D., P. M. O'Malley et al. (2003). Monitoring the Future national survey results on drug use, 1975-2003: Volume 1, Secondary school students. Bethesda, MD: National Institute on Drug Abuse.

Kroll, J., M. Habenicht et al. (1989). "Depression and posttraumatic stress disorder in Southeast Asian refugees." *American Journal of Psychiatry* 146(12): 1592-7.

Kuramoto, F. H. (1995). "Asian and Pacific Island community alcohol prevention research." *Challenge of Participatory Research: Preventing Alcohol-related Problems in Ethnic Communities.* P. A. Langton, L. G. Epstein, and M. A. Orlandi, Center for Substance Abuse Prevention: 411-428.

Lai, M. (2003). "The status of Oakland's API youth: Findings from the interim report." *apiCurrents* 3(1): 2-3.

Le, T. (2001). Not invisible: Asian Pacific Islander juvenile arrests in Alameda County. Oakland, CA: National Council on Crime and Delinquency: Asian/Pacific Islander Youth Violence Prevention Center.

Miyares, I. M. (1998). *The Hmong Refugee Experience in America: Crossing the River.* New York: Garland Publishing, Inc.

NCCD (2003). Under the microscope: Asian and Pacific Islander youth in Oakland. Oakland, CA: National Council on Crime and Delinquency: Asian/Pacific Islander Youth Violence Prevention Center.

NCCD (n.d.). Asian and Pacific Islander youth in West Contra Costa County. Oakland, CA, National Council on Crime and Delinquency: Asian/Pacific Islander Youth Violence Prevention Center (unpublished report).

Ngor, H. S., and R. Warner (1987). *A Cambodian Odyssey*. New York: Macmillan Publishing Company.

Nicassio, P. M. (1985). "The psychosocial adjustment of the Southeast Asian refugee: An overview of empirical findings and theoretical models." *Journal of Cross-Cultural Psychology* 16(2): 153-173.

O'Hare, T. ,and T. Van Tran (1998). "Substance abuse among Southeast Asians in the U.S.: Implications for practice and research." *Social Work in Health Care* 26(3).

Parker, H., J. Aldridge et al. (1998). *Illegal Leisure: The Normalization of Adolescent Recreational Drug Use*. London and New York: Routledge.

Perkins, W. E. (Ed.) (1996). *Droppin' Science: Critical Essays on Rap Music and Hip Hop Culture*. Philadelphia: Temple University Press.

Portes, A., and R. G. Rumbaut (2001). *Legacies: The Story of the Immigrant Second Generation*. Berkeley, CA: University of California Press.

Ross, A. and T. Rose, Eds. (1994). *Microphone Fiends: Youth Music Youth Culture*. New York, Routledge.

Saecho, F. L., Ed. (n.d., ca. 1999). *Quietly Torn: A literary journal by Iu Mien American youth*. San Francisco, CA: Pacific News Service.

Szymusiak, M. (1999). *The Stones Cry Out; A Cambodian Childhood 1975-1980*. Bloomington, IN: Indiana University Press.

Unger, J. B., T. B. Cruz et al. (2000). "English language use as a risk factor for smoking initiation among Hispanic and Asian American adolescents: Evidence for mediation by tobacco-related beliefs and social norms." *Health Psychology* 19(5): 403-410.

Urberg, K. A., S. M. Degirmencioglu et al. (2000). "Adolescent social crowds: Measurement and relationship to friendships." *Journal of Adolescent Research* 15(4): 427-445.

Waters, T. (1999). *Crime and Immigrant Youth*. Thousand Oaks, CA: Sage Publications.

Westermeyer, J. (1988). "Sex differences in drug and alcohol use among ethnic groups in Laos, 1965-1975." *American Journal of Drug and Alcohol Abuse* 14(4): 443-461.

Westermeyer, J., T. Lyfoung et al. (1989). "An epidemic of opium dependence among Asian refugees in Minnesota: Characteristics and causes." *British Journal of Addiction* 84(7): 785-789.

Westermeyer, J., T. Lyfoung et al. (1991). "Opium addiction among Indochinese refugees in the United States: Characteristics of addicts and their opium use." *American Journal of Drug Alcohol Abuse* 17(3): 267-77.

Yee, B. W., and N. D. Thu (1987). "Correlates of drug use and abuse among Indochinese refugees: Mental health implications." *Journal of Psychoactive Drugs* 19(1).

# Using Marijuana in Adulthood:
# The Experience of a Sample of Users
# in Oklahoma City

Rashi K. Shukla, PhD

**SUMMARY.** This study examines marijuana involvement among a sample of adult users in Oklahoma City, Oklahoma. Semi-structured interviews were conducted with 29 adult marijuana users between 2000 and 2002. Qualitative analyses of data on patterns of marijuana involvement in adulthood were conducted. Marijuana use is a leisure-time activity users engage in with close peers or alone. Adult users limit their consumption of marijuana to free time, and keep their marijuana use from interfering with other responsibilities. These adult users are controlled marijuana users; they view their involvement with marijuana as a personal, private, recreational activity. *[Article copies available for a fee from The Haworth Document Delivery Service: 1-800-HAWORTH. E-mail address: <docdelivery@haworthpress.com> Website: <http://www.HaworthPress.com> © 2005 by The Haworth Press, Inc. All rights reserved.]*

**KEYWORDS.** Adult, marijuana use, marijuana involvement, adulthood

---

Rashi K. Shukla is Assistant Professor of Criminal Justice, University of Central Oklahoma, Department of Sociology, Criminal Justice and Substance Abuse Studies, 100 North University Drive, Edmond, OK 73034 (E-mail: rshukla@ucok.edu).

[Haworth co-indexing entry note]: "Using Marijuana in Adulthood: The Experience of a Sample of Users in Oklahoma City." Shukla, Rashi K. Co-published simultaneously in *Journal of Ethnicity in Substance Abuse* (The Haworth Press, Inc.) Vol. 4, No. 3/4, 2005, pp. 153-181; and: *The Cultural/Subcultural Contexts of Marijuana Use at the Turn of the Twenty-First Century* (ed: Andrew Golub) The Haworth Press, Inc., 2005, pp. 153-181. Single or multiple copies of this article are available for a fee from The Haworth Document Delivery Service [1-800-HAWORTH, 9:00 a.m. - 5:00 p.m. (EST). E-mail address: docdelivery@haworthpress.com].

doi:10.1300/J233v04n03_07

## INTRODUCTION

Studies that have examined illicit drug use among users heavily immersed in a drug-using or criminal lifestyle (see Biernacki, 1986; Bourgois, 2003; Lindesmith, 1968; Sterk, 1999; Williams, 1989) have focused on populations with drug use patterns that are very different from illicit drug use among users who remain tied to conventional roles and responsibilities (see Parker, Aldridge & Measham, 1998; Waldorf, Reinarman & Murphy, 1991) or who are controlled drug users (Zinberg, 1984; Zinberg, Harding, & Winkeller, 1977). To the extent that subcultures and drug users are heterogeneous, differences in types of users and levels of involvement with drug use and the drug-using lifestyle must be taken into consideration. The heterogeneity that exists among drug users is evident even among hard drug users. In research with heroin and non-opiate drug users, Sutter (1970) described the heterogeneous culture of street drug users as one that is composed of "different types of drug users, different sets of practices, different life styles and perspectives" (p. 83). Such variations are likely to be evident both among users of a single type of drug, as well as among different types of drug users. There is a need to develop a greater understanding of variations among drug users in terms of different patterns of use and level of immersion in a drug-using lifestyle.

This study examines the marijuana use experience of a sample of adult users. Data from qualitative interviews provide insight into how marijuana use as a social activity changes in adulthood, and how these adult users accommodate marijuana into their lifestyles. The research presented here describes a sample of illicit drug users (i.e., marijuana) who live conventional lifestyles. The users in the current study are likely to be very different from the types of illicit drug users described in studies of users immersed in a drug-using lifestyle.

## LITERATURE REVIEW

### The Drug-Immersed Lifestyle

Detailed descriptions of the lifestyles of individuals immersed in a life associated with illicit drugs have emerged from ethnographies of cocaine users and dealers (see Adler, 1993; Bourgois, 2003; Sterk, 1999; Williams, 1989). These ethnographies have provided a qualitative understanding of the conflicts and struggles faced by individuals heavily involved in a lifestyle intertwined with illicit drugs. Individuals immersed in a drug lifestyle lead lives tightly connected to the world of illicit drug use. Their social relationships and daily activities are heavily influenced by their involvement with illicit drugs. To the extent that their lives revolve around dealing and using illicit drugs, their involvement with pro-social, conventional activities is minimized.

In *The Cocaine Kids*, Williams (1989) describes the lifestyles of eight teenage cocaine dealers. Documenting their journeys in the world of cocaine, Williams illustrates how the lifestyles of these young people are influenced by their involvement with cocaine. In their lives, their work, peers, and leisure-time activities are all related to cocaine; they live a lifestyle that distinguishes them from more conventional members of society. Constantly hustling and working to make money and maintain their position in the cocaine ring, the lives of the youth in Williams' study revolve around cocaine. Within this subculture, the lines between using and dealing often become blurred. Young cocaine dealers often go through periods of time when their own consumption of cocaine gets out of control and threatens their ability to maintain their cocaine dealing. With access to money, weapons and cocaine, the youth in *The Cocaine Kids* struggle to balance their involvement in the cocaine trade with the other roles and responsibilities they maintain. During the period of time in which the youth live lives immersed in dealing and using cocaine, their involvement with conventional activities such as legitimate work and going to school are viewed as being of secondary importance to their drug-related activities. What is particularly interesting about *The Cocaine Kids* are the changes they experience by the end of the study when they begin to reach adulthood. As the teenagers get older, the cocaine market begins to change and become more dangerous. They begin to understand that continued involvement with the cocaine trade is becoming increasingly risky. They start to see a conflict between their ability to stay involved in cocaine dealing and their movement into a more normal life. As a result, even these youth who were once heavily immersed in the world of cocaine see the temporary nature of their involvement in a lifestyle that revolves around the cocaine market. They understand that they have a choice to make–cocaine dealing, or a conventional life. In the end, the tragedies and risks associated with immersion in the world of cocaine take their toll on *The Kids*. By the time they enter young adulthood, "those who had a stake in something" (p. 131), be it school, family, or something else, left the life of cocaine trafficking for more conventional lives.

## Limited Drug Involvement and Maturation

While not all individuals immersed in the drug-using lifestyle leave the lifestyle, the observed patterns of change experienced by *The Cocaine Kids* as they entered adulthood are not unique. Although *The Cocaine Kids* differ from other illicit drug users in a number of ways (e.g., they were heavily involved in dealing cocaine), for most people involvement with illicit drug use changes over time. In one of the first studies to document reductions in involvement with drug use among addicts, Winick (1962) coined the term *maturation* to refer to observed termination of involvement with illicit drug use in adulthood. In his study of known narcotic addicts, Winick (1962) found that a number of addicts became inactive in their thirties. Follow-up studies with other populations of drug addicts have confirmed the existence of maturation among at least some individuals who use illicit drugs (see Ball & Snarr, 1969; Snow, 1973). A majority of illicit drug users eventually stop using drugs in adulthood (Bachman, Wadsworth, O'Malley, Johnston, & Schulenberg, 1997; Chen & Kandel, 1995; Kandel & Logan, 1984; Kandel & Raveis, 1989; Kandel, Yamaguchi &, Chen, 1992; Labouvie, 1996). Researchers have sought to understand why such changes occur. Explanations for the observed reductions in illicit drug use include: changes in personal development (Labouvie, 1996), new adult roles and living arrangements (Bachman et al., 1997), reductions in time spent with peers after marriage (Warr, 1998), changing perceptions of risks and disapproval (Bachman et al., 2002), and a lack of interest (Cohen & Kaal, 2001) in drug use.

A descriptive pattern of typical involvement with illicit drug use has emerged from studies of drug use. Involvement with marijuana and other illicit drugs peaks in adolescence and young adulthood and decreases over time (Johnston, O'Malley, & Bachman, 2001; Kandel & Logan, 1984; Merline, O'Malley, Schulenberg, Bachman, & Johnston, 2004). Most of the young people who initiate illicit drugs do not "use them to excess" (Bachman et al., 1997, p. 1); they experiment with illicit substances without becoming regular users. For most, involvement with illicit drug use resembles a temporary phase. Individuals experiment with or use illicit drugs for a limited period of time (Bachman et al., 1997; Labouvie, 1996; Labouvie & White, 2002) and then stop. While this represents the typical pattern of involvement with illicit drug use, not all individuals stop using illicit substances in adulthood. Some illicit drug users continue using illicit substances (e.g., marijuana) in adulthood. Little is known about adults who use illicit substances within the context of their otherwise conventional life. These are the users of interest here.

## The Most Commonly Used Illicit Drug

Marijuana use serves as the focus of the present study because it is the most commonly used illicit drug (Office of National Drug Control Policy [ONDCP], 2004; Substance Abuse and Mental Health Services Administration [SAMSHA], 2003, 2004). High rates of marijuana use have been found in samples of the general population (SAMSHA, 2003, 2004), high school students (Johnston, O'Malley, Bachman & Schulenberg, 2004) and jail populations (Golub & Johnson, 2001; National Institute of Justice [NIJ], 1999). Although the exact number of adult users cannot be precisely determined (see Becker, 1963; Earlywine, 2002; Goode, 1970), estimates of current users at any given time range in the millions. According to recent findings from the National Survey on Drug Use and Health (NSDUH), 4.8 million of the estimated 25.8 million Americans age 12 and older who used marijuana in the past year "reported using marijuana 20 or more days in the past month" (ONDCP, 2004, p. 1). A recent follow-up survey of Monitoring the Future participants at age 35 found that 13% of men and 7% of women reported using marijuana in the past 30 days (Merline et al., 2004). Marijuana has been identified as the drug of choice among illicit drug users in both the arrestee (NIJ, 2000) and general populations (Golub & Johnson, 2001; Golub, Johnson, Dunlap, & Sifaneck, 2004). Yet, few studies have specifically examined the marijuana experiences of adult users. This is a critical gap in the literature. In a recent report on cannabis by the Canadian Senate Special Committee on Illegal Drugs (Canada, Parliament, 2003), the Committee found, "few sociological or anthropological studies are conducted on the circumstances or context of illegal drug use, specifically for cannabis . . . the result is that our pool of knowledge on users and characteristics of use is sorely lacking" (p. 44). While national surveys such as the National Household Survey on Drug Use and Health (SAMSHA, 2003, 2004), Monitoring the Future (Johnston et al., 2004), and Arrestee Drug Abuse Monitoring Program (NIJ, 2003) provide estimates on the prevalence of marijuana involvement within the populations surveyed, these studies do not provide in-depth, contextual information on patterns of marijuana involvement among adult users.

## Marijuana Users

Within the social sciences, a number of researchers have sought to gain an insider's perspective of marijuana involvement (see Becker, 1953, 1963; Goode, 1970; Zinberg, 1984). In one of the earliest studies of marijuana use, Becker (1953, 1963) sought to explain "the use of marihuana for pleasure" (1963, p. 43). According to Becker, an individual will use marijuana for pleasure when he or she learns the technique of smoking marijuana, learns to experience the effects associated with the use of marijuana, and learns to enjoy the experience. Becker focused on users within the culture of the dance musician and found that members of this group differed from others to such a degree that they were "a group of 'outsiders' that considered themselves and were considered by others to be 'different'" (Becker, 1963, p. 101). By examining how deviant subcultures behave, view themselves, and respond to external pressures, Becker's research laid the foundation for future studies of marijuana use and the subcultures of individuals who use marijuana. In a later study of marijuana users, Goode (1970) expanded on the variations that exist between marijuana users by presenting a typology of different categories of users, including experimenters, occasional users, regular users and frequent users. Goode also noted that the perspectives of users often differed from outside perspectives on marijuana use, and linked the many misconceptions and myths about marijuana use to the moral and stereotypical views often associated with marijuana users (Goode, 1970). Goode reiterated the need for researchers to continue to study marijuana use, arguing:

> Marijuana use today is not a fad, not a craze. It is not going to be wished away and legal measures to eradicate it will be only partially successful. Whether we like it or not, pot smoking is here to stay. It might be wise to try to understand it. (p. 4)

These words are as relevant today as they were back in 1970. While both Becker and Goode acknowledged the problems associated with studying marijuana due to its hidden nature and illegality, they also understood the potential contributions that social research on marijuana involvement could make.

## Changing Context

The context in which marijuana use occurs today is quite different than when Becker (1953, 1963) and Goode (1970) conducted their studies. Although the United States is in the midst of a War on Drugs against illicit drugs including marijuana, attitudes about the criminalization of marijuana are shifting (Canada, Parliament, 2003). References to marijuana appear in the media (ONDCP, 2002), on television shows, and in movies and song lyrics. There are pro-marijuana groups (e.g., NORML) and subcultures of users with new methods of consumption (e.g., blunts) (Golub & Johnson, 1999). There is even evidence that the purity and potency of marijuana is changing (Drug Enforcement Administration [DEA], 2003). Within this changing context, marijuana continues to be both a subcultural and a social activity. It is subcultural to the extent that the individuals who use it are likely to share certain attitudes and behaviors in common, and are thus differentiated from non-users (Becker, 1963; Brake, 1980; Cloward & Ohlin, 1960; Goode, 1970). Marijuana use is social in that users often prefer to share the use experience with other users (Goode, 1970; McCambridge & Strang, 2004; National Commission on Marihuana & Drug Abuse, 1972).

Two replications of Becker's original research (Hallstone, 2002; Hirsch, Conforti, & Graney, 1990) have contributed to our understanding of historical and contextual changes in the marijuana-using scene. Though conducted with two geographically different populations of marijuana users (i.e., Wisconsin and Hawaii), both replications found that Becker's stages of involvement were still applicable. However, the replications supported the idea that the marijuana-using scene is changing. In both studies, the majority of respondents became intoxicated, reported getting high, and indicated that they enjoyed their first experience with marijuana (Hallstone, 2002; Hirsch et al., 1990). In explaining these findings, the researchers pointed to historical changes in the marijuana using scene, particularly the more mainstream nature of marijuana use today (Hallstone, 2002), and to changes in cultural attitudes and smoking technologies (Hirsch et al., 1990).

There is also evidence that a new era of drug users referred to as the Marijuana Blunts Generation are coming through the criminal justice system (Golub & Johnson, 1999). Arrestees in this cohort of individuals prefer to use marijuana in the form of a blunt over other illicit drugs, and are less likely to progress to other forms of illicit drug use than previous generations of arrestees in the Manhattan criminal justice system. In comparing the marijuana involvement of these arrestees (i.e., ADAM) with individuals in the general population (i.e., NHSDA), Golub et al. (2004) found that the arrestees were more likely to continue using marijuana throughout their twenties than users in the general population. These divergent patterns of involvement suggest that a greater understanding of differences in patterns of marijuana involvement among different types of users is necessary.

## Patterns of Use

Not all individuals who use illicit drugs are drug addicts. There exists a misconception that all illicit drug users use drugs compulsively and are involved in various criminal behaviors. For individuals who use marijuana, some level of involvement in illegal behavior is inevitable due to the fact that the behaviors related to possessing and acquiring marijuana are illegal. However, involvement with marijuana does not require immersion in a criminal lifestyle. Many individuals who use marijuana do so without being involved in other criminal or deviant behaviors. Only a small proportion of individuals who use marijuana become problem users of the drug (Earlywine, 2002; Goldstein, 2001; Mack & Joy, 2001); marijuana use has not been found to be detrimental for the majority of users (Mack & Joy, 2001).

Researchers have found that the typical pattern of marijuana use is casual and recreational (Becker, 1963; Goode, 1970; Zinberg, 1984). Becker (1963) was the first to point this out:

> Marihuana does not produce addiction, at least in the sense that alcohol and the opiate drugs do. The user experiences no withdrawal sickness and exhibits no ineradicable craving for the drug . . . the drug is used occasionally for the pleasure the user finds in it, a relatively casual kind of behavior in comparison with that connected with the use of addicting drugs. (p. 43)

Similarly, Goode (1970) challenged the stereotypical view of marijuana users as individuals who are high all day, every day, finding the *recreational model* of use to be most accurate. Together, these findings support the noncompulsive, episodic nature of marijuana use. While there are individuals who use marijuana compulsively and become problem users of the drug (see Stephens, Roffman, & Simpson, 1993; Weiner, Sussman, McCullen, William, & Lichtman, 1999), the evidence suggests that these users may be the exception rather than the norm. In a recent review of the scientific literature on marijuana, Earlywine (2002) reiterated what is known about marijuana:

> A few points about marijuana remain unarguable . . . Recreational use has (also) been around for thousands of years. Cannabis is the

most popular illicit drug in the world. Hundreds of millions of people have tried it. Only a small fraction of them develop problems with other illicit drugs. Less than one-tenth of the people who ever try marijuana end up using it regularly. Fewer still develop troubles with it. (p. 271)

## The Study

This study examines the marijuana involvement of an adult sample of users in Oklahoma City, Oklahoma. Specifically, this study explores how adult marijuana users integrate their marijuana use into their otherwise conventional lifestyles. The experience of marijuana use in adulthood is described from the perspective of the adult users. Data are presented on the nature of marijuana use as a social activity in adulthood. This paper contributes to what is known about patterns of marijuana use in adulthood by focusing specifically on a sample of adult users who are tied to conventional society. A majority of them are employed; they are all involved in conventional activities. To the extent that the users in this study are invested in and tied to conventional society, it can be argued that they have a lot to lose if their marijuana use is detected (see Golub et al., 2004). This paper describes how the adult users in this study accommodate marijuana use into their life, and the types of informal rules users adhere to, to keep their use from being detected, from becoming problematic, and from interfering in their lives.

## METHODS

The data used in this study were compiled as part of a larger, exploratory, qualitative study on marijuana use and decision-making (see Shukla, 2003). Qualitative methods are based on a different set of assumptions about the research process (Maxwell, 1996; Neuman & Weigand, 2000) and are especially suited for studies where little is known; they allow for the collection of in-depth, contextual information on the topic of interest, in this case, marijuana use. In the present study, the research process incorporated both deduction and induction (Babbie, 2005). During the early stages of the research, a deductive approach was taken. Initially, the aim of the study was to explore the utility of examining illicit drug use from a decision-making perspective. As a result, the study was designed with the rational choice perspective (Clarke &

Cornish, 2001, 1985; Cornish & Clarke, 1986) as a framework; initial sampling considerations and the interview instrument were influenced by the assumptions and general framework of the rational choice perspective. However, given the overall goal of gaining a grounded understanding of decision-making and drug use (i.e., versus hypothesis testing), flexibility was maintained throughout the research process. Specific research questions and the analytical focus evolved as the data were collected. In the later stages of the research, an inductive approach based on grounded theory (Charmaz & Mitchell, 2001; Glaser & Strauss, 1967; Strauss & Corbin, 1998) guided the data collection and analyses. Broader themes, patterns, and analytical codes were grounded in, and emerged from the data.

A purposive (Schwandt, 1997), theoretical (Glaser & Strauss, 1967; Strauss & Corbin, 1998) sampling strategy using snowball sampling (Biernacki & Waldorf, 1981) techniques was used to identify both current and ex-users of marijuana. Given the initial focus of the study, individuals with a range of past and present experiences with marijuana were determined to be theoretically relevant. While the initial sampling strategy called for locating and interviewing 50 subjects, sampling decisions were based on theoretical considerations. All subjects were a minimum of 18 years old. Sampling began with the identification of a three key informants with ties to marijuana users. Through snowball sampling, individuals were referred to the study for participation either by the key informants or through other subjects. Subjects were interviewed if they met the criteria of being either a regular or ex-user of marijuana. This was determined by asking subjects "Have you ever used marijuana?" Subjects were then asked if they were current users or ex-users of marijuana for further classification. Data from ex-users of marijuana are excluded from this analysis.

### The Sample

The data presented here are based on interviews with 29 adult marijuana users. These subjects all answered "Yes" to the question "Do you currently use marijuana?" Subjects were self-identified as 19 regular marijuana users and 10 social users of marijuana. They ranged in level of use from daily use (n = 14), to using marijuana multiple times a week (n = 13) and multiple times a year (n = 2). The subjects in this study had marijuana use careers ranging from one year to thirty-four years. Use career was calculated by comparing age of initiation with the current age of the subject. Periodic breaks in the use of marijuana were not accounted for in calculating the length of marijuana use career. The average marijuana use career for the individuals in this study is 16 years.

The sample includes 17 males and 12 females; twenty-five of the subjects are Caucasian. They range in age from 18 to 52 years old. The average age of subjects is 31 years old. The adults in this study are unique in that the majority of them are college-educated and employed. Of the 29 subjects, 27 of them are legitimately employed in various types of jobs from service or manual labor to employment within a professional occupation. Nineteen of the subjects have some college or higher, including 5 individuals who have one or more graduate degrees. The majority of subjects (n = 18) in this study have not had contact with the criminal justice system. With few exceptions, individuals with prior arrests (n = 11) were arrested primarily for minor criminal offenses (e.g., possession, a DUI) related to their drug use. In the presentation of the data, pseudonyms are being used to protect the anonymity of the subjects.

Data were collected in Oklahoma City, Oklahoma between 2000 and 2002. Retrospective interviews were utilized as the primary data collection method. The interviews were face-to-face interviews conducted in person, in various public places (e.g., restaurants, bars, etc.). Interviews were audio-taped and then transcribed. The average interview lasted one hour. The interview instrument consisted of approximately 100 semi-structured, open-ended questions. The specific interview questions were structured with the rational choice perspective (Clarke & Cornish, 2001, 1985; Cornish & Clarke, 1986) as a framework. Questions were asked about the following topics: decision-making processes associated with initiation, continuation, and desistance from marijuana use, past and current drug use, patterns of drug use, and thoughts about future drug use. The questions were designed to gain the individuals' own perspectives on their drug experiences. Informed consent was obtained from each subject prior to participation. Respondents were paid $10 compensation. The qualitative software program askSam™ was used to assist with data coding and management. Codes were inductively generated and attached to the data. A constant comparative method was used to identify themes and patterns in the data (Glaser & Strauss, 1967). The findings that follow are based on analyses of interview data bits where individuals discussed marijuana involvement in adulthood as it related to leisure activities, lifestyles, and peers.

The findings in this study are limited to the degree that they are based on self-report data from a small sample of adults in Oklahoma City. The sample is predominantly white and middle-class. The majority of them are college-educated and employed. This population is likely to be very different from populations of individuals heavily enmeshed in drug-using or criminal lifestyles. To the extent that the subjects in this study are not representative of all marijuana users, the findings have limited generalizability. In light of the exploratory purpose of understanding patterns of marijuana use in adulthood, generalizability is not the goal. The marijuana use experiences of the adults in this study, however, may be similar to other marijuana-using adults who lead primarily conventional lives.

### Drug Histories

The drug histories of the individuals in this study put their current marijuana use in context. A majority of the individuals in this sample had drug histories that involved the use of illicit drugs other than marijuana. The two subjects with the fewest past experiences with other illicit drugs admitted only to inhaling legal substances (e.g., liquid paper) experimentally. All of the subjects had histories of involvement with legal substances (i.e., alcohol, tobacco). A few individuals discussed periods of problematic drug use in the past, and only two of the marijuana users had ever attended a drug treatment program for their drug use. At the time of the interview, both of these subjects were using marijuana and did not feel that their use was problematic. Three of the younger subjects in the study were different from the others in that they described themselves as being in a temporary phase of drug use. They indicated that they were using a number of different illicit substances and were likely to continue to initiate and use illicit substances other than marijuana. What is interesting is that even these three subjects, who were in their late teens and early twenties, described their current level of illicit drug use as temporary, and something that they plan to stop when they get older and begin to take on more adult responsibilities. Although subjects varied with regard to level of past drug use in terms of the frequency of other illicit drug use and the total number of other illicit substances ever used, all of the subjects had experienced reductions in illicit drug involvement over time. At the time of the interview, the majority of subjects were only using legal substances (i.e., alcohol and/or tobacco) and marijuana. Only a few of the adult marijuana users indicated that they might consider using an illicit substance other than marijuana (e.g., mushrooms) on rare occasions (e.g., once every few years).

# FINDINGS

## Question #1: To what extent is marijuana use in adulthood a social activity?

Marijuana use as a social activity changes in adulthood. The majority of adult users stated that they preferred using marijuana with others. Adult users discussed enjoying the social experience of "getting high" and using marijuana with other users, particularly close friends or family members. Mark, a 33-year old marijuana user, explained his preference for using marijuana socially:

> I easily prefer it in the company of friends . . . 'Cuz I think it's a social drug, I really do . . . with marijuana it's almost like it *entices* you to be social to some degree, you know, you *want* to talk to people, you want to find out ways to do different things, how people are doing, but I do think that a lot of that too has to do with that relaxed mental state that you're put into, because I don't think we as a people have, I don't think we get into a relaxed mental state very often.

Other users shared similar sentiments about the benefits of sharing the marijuana use experience. Kara, a 24-year-old marijuana user, described why she views marijuana to be a social drug:

> Well, I just know, that like, a lot of the, people . . . they consider it, that, that it's a *gift, you share*, and you know, want to be around other people and (it makes) you laugh at the things with everybody, you know, just, *experience the same things, together*, you know what I'm sayin'?

Although most users preferred using marijuana socially, patterns of marijuana use in adulthood are influenced by declines in the number of the users' friends who continue to use marijuana. While all of the users knew other people who still used marijuana, the number of their peers who continued to use it in adulthood had decreased over time. As a result of these changes in marijuana involvement among their peers, adult users become more willing and likely to use marijuana alone. The decline in marijuana use among friends was a common theme throughout the interviews. Adult marijuana users appreciated and understood why their peers, who were once marijuana users themselves, might stop using marijuana in adulthood, Mark explains:

> Sometimes other people, because they have *changes in their life*, will stop doing, you know, certain things, I mean if you're a breast-feeding mother, you know, and, and for, for most of my friends, that's respected, you know, you're not, 'well you always used to smoke pot, just 'cuz you have a kid you're going to stop smoking pot?' You know, most of the time its 'hell yes, I'm going to stop smoking pot because I have a kid' you know, it's illegal, and DHS (Department of Human Services) could come in here, the neighbors report me, and take my child away because of what a horrible parent I am.

Leeza, a 47-year-old marijuana user, similarly noted the decline in use among her peers:

> I probably know maybe three, four, five people, they probably use (marijuana) regularly, and then most of the other people I know use it, just use it you know, occasionally, or at a party. [Do you use marijuana mostly alone or with other people?] Alone, 'cuz I don't know anybody to do it with, unless I go visit Steven (a friend who also uses marijuana).

Having been a regular marijuana user for over 20 years, Leeza expanded on the significant decrease in number of peers who continue to use marijuana as time passes:

> Very few, as time goes on. Especially, I had one friend who uses it, she only used it . . . when she can get it, but she's not a regular user. I have other friends . . . they probably use it socially, I mean if somebody passed it to them at a party they'd probably take a hit, um, I only have one or two friends that are like me, that use it on a regular, well Steven is one, a friend that I've known for a long time, he's a regular user.

Reductions in marijuana use among peers were not restricted to older subjects. Although in her early twenties at the time of the interview, Kara had already witnessed a significant reduction in the number of her peers who used marijuana:

> That I know . . . definitely a minority, definitely now, 'cuz they're
> all, like I said, married, have kids, professional. [Have most of
> them quit using drugs?] I think so, the, the people I grew up with,
> just the responsibilities, it was like you know, just grew out of it.
> [Do you use marijuana mostly alone or with other people?] Proba-
> bly mostly alone now, because so few, you know, people do it any-
> more.

Only T.J., a 50-year-old marijuana user, described having a preference
to use marijuana alone that had nothing to do with changes in use among
his peers:

> If I use it (now), and it's pretty rare, I use it alone so I can listen to
> music . . . I really don't care for the high anymore and I don't do it
> very often, just every once in awhile I'll decide I want to. I don't
> like to do it with other people, I like, I like to get some kind of per-
> cussion album, maybe Mozart or something, just anything, you
> know I'll want to hear this piece of music high and I'll get it, that's
> the only reason I ever want to do it (anymore) . . .

For some, reductions in leisure time spent with friends who used marijuana also influenced patterns of marijuana use in adulthood. Ely, a
32-year-old user, described this here:

> I don't hang around with people who smoke it as much now as I
> used to, I mean used to I'd be around people like daily that, you
> know were waiting to smoke it and now, I pretty much go to work
> and come home. We don't smoke it at (band) practice you know,
> so I end up smoking it, like if I'm on my way to, to something, um,
> you know, but yeah.

There is also evidence that the influence of peers' marijuana use on
individual marijuana use decreases in adulthood. The majority of adult
marijuana users talked about making decisions about marijuana use on
the basis of whether they felt like using it, rather than whether or not
their peers were using it. In comparison to marijuana use during adolescence which is highly peer-related, the situational influence of peers'
use decreases in adulthood. This is illustrated by Mark's description of
the situational context in which he uses marijuana today:

> If I had to define it, I'd probably say it's regular because I don't do it just strictly in a social situation with other people, um, I would do it in, *in fact, it's rare*, I don't think it has much to do anymore with the situation as far as being around friends or anything like that. It's more like my mental state at that point. I have gone to parties before, and not smoked any, you know, just because I wasn't into it.

For the adult marijuana users in this study, marijuana use continues to be a social, but not strictly social behavior. While many adult users prefer using marijuana with close friends or family, changes in patterns of marijuana use in adulthood are influenced by changes in the number of peers who continue to use marijuana in adulthood, reductions in leisure time spent with other users, and changes in the influence peers have on use itself. Adults who continue using marijuana in adulthood adapt to these changes by becoming more willing and likely to use marijuana alone. Adult users tend to make decisions about marijuana use on the basis of whether or not they feel like using it, rather than on the basis of whether their peers are using marijuana.

### Question #2: How does marijuana use fit into the lifestyle of the adults in this study?

Adult life is very different from life during adolescence. Adulthood brings with it new roles and responsibilities. Lifestyles change as leisure time decreases and people become increasingly involved in maintaining their adult roles and responsibilities. The individuals in this study provided a unique picture of how marijuana use fits into the context of their primarily conventional lifestyles. When viewed within this context, it is evident that their marijuana use is a recreational activity of secondary importance to the conventional roles and responsibilities they maintain. Marijuana use is placed behind other, more important life considerations such as work and family responsibilities. The users in this study provided insight on how their involvement with marijuana use fits into their lifestyles, and on the norms, or informal rules, they adhere to, to keep their marijuana use from interfering with other aspects of their life.

Marijuana use is a recreational, leisure activity users engage in only when they have free time. The majority of adult users indicated that their level of marijuana use continuously changes and varies over time. They discussed increasing or decreasing the frequency of their marijuana use depending on other factors in their life. Andrea, a 36-year-old marijuana user, described how her frequency of marijuana use changes over time depending on other life considerations:

> It varies, depending on what I have going on. If I'm doing a lot of writing, then, more of my leisure time involves drugs (marijuana only). But then, it's also common, for me to go over to my friends' house, and we'll sit around and get stoned and talk, and, so I mean, how much of my time? I can't tell you specifically in terms of hours. It depends on what I'm doing, again. It can be a lot of my time during the week, or it can be, none of my time during the week. If I'm doing something creative, then, drugs are likely to be employed, or marijuana is.

All of the adult marijuana users indicated that they stopped using marijuana during times when they had other things to do or didn't want to use. Variations in frequency of marijuana use were often related to changes in life circumstances. For example, Stacy is a 21-year-old marijuana user who stated that she is currently using marijuana more frequently than usual because she is temporarily unemployed. Here, she discusses her level of use when she's working regularly:

> Um, *recreationally*, three or four times a week, at best, um, I was *workin' a lot*, because *I don't do it at work*, so, I wasn't *buyin' it*, it was, be more like, if I saw a friend after work, and they had it, so, yeah, more social, recreationally.

She was adamant that the frequency of her use would decrease once she began working again. She explains:

> Like *right now*, I'm in between jobs, and, my . . . and my *drug use*, has gone *up*, 'cuz I have more free time, 'cuz I don't, *I don't use it when I go to work*, or when I have things I have to, be *responsible* for, so, that's 8 hours of my day, that's 8 hours of my day that, *I have*, so, right, so now, I don't have a job, so I can do whatever I want.

Similar sentiments regarding changes in one's frequency and level of marijuana use were shared by others as well. While a few individuals talked about going through phases in their life when they were younger where they were heavy marijuana users, using marijuana all day long or multiple times a day every day, this pattern of use did not characterize the marijuana involvement of the adult users in this sample. Adult marijuana users were adamant about keeping their marijuana involvement separate from other areas of their lives (e.g., work). They consciously do not use marijuana when they have to work, or have other obligations and responsibilities to attend to. This is something Tom, a 31-year-old user, was resolute about. On how his marijuana use fits into his lifestyle he explained:

> Social life, recreationally in my social life, that's the only way it fits in. I don't, it has nothing to do with my job, nor do I go to work or perform on my job, under the influence of marijuana, ever. [You function normally and get everything you need done?] Absolutely. [Does your marijuana use interfere with anything?] No, I don't let it. Yeah, I mean, it's a de-motivator, to take care of tasks, I will say for sure, so I mean, I don't, I consciously don't do it if I have something that I know it's going to make me not want to do or prevent me from doing. But I mean, I don't use it in the mornings, and I don't, ever use while I'm at work, and you know, occasionally when I come home from work, and on the weekends.

Tom described the self-imposed rules that regulate the context in which he uses marijuana:

> I don't use it on my job, I, I use it when I'm playing, in the band, but I don't do it on stage or you know, I do it beforehand. [Have you ever missed work because of your marijuana use?] Oh no, no, I make it, it, it fits into areas of my life where there's not anything, you know, it's a free-time thing.

These adult marijuana users consume marijuana only in their free time. They purposely do not use marijuana when they have other things to do. They make an important distinction between the activities they engage in during their leisure time and the other responsibilities they have.

None of the adult users in this study believed that their marijuana use interfered with their life in any significant way. While all acknowledged the potential risks of being involved with marijuana as an illegal drug, they engaged in a number of self-regulatory strategies to minimize the potential risks of their continued involvement with marijuana. These strategies include not using marijuana when they have other things to do, keeping their use low-key and hidden from certain people in their lives, and purposely limiting their consumption of marijuana. Although the actual risks of being arrested for using or possessing marijuana were relatively low for the individuals in this study, they were nonetheless very cognizant of the risks associated with their on-going marijuana consumption. Leeza, a 47-year-old mother who uses marijuana, discussed the risks of her use and how they've changed over time:

> I think as time has gone on, in this decade it's been more of a problem just 'cuz I've really had to, you know become more clandestine, like I would *never* smoke it in my car or have it in my car. You know, the times that I go get it and I drive back home, you know it always seems like I see a police car, and it's just like 'God' you know. I think it's impacted my life that way, the Drug War, and you know the kids, they go through the DARE program, unless you specifically request for them to opt out, and I don't want to do that. I don't want them to be targeted in anyway, or wonder why, yeah, and it seems to slide off their backs anyway.

She talked about the conflict of being a marijuana-using mother who hides her use from her children. While she made the decision not to tell her children about her use, she worried about what would happen if they ever found out:

> I don't want to come out of the closet to my kids, as a doper (marijuana user), so, if the subject comes up, and I feel fairly safe saying don't do LSD, and since I have daughters I try to say, and I really haven't touched on it or lectured them, but when the subject comes up, I'll be like you know you shouldn't try any illegal drug, or any drug, when you're young. You know I say when you're an adult, if you make the decision to try something that's fine, as long as you don't have a problem with it, but you know when you're in school and your life is all ahead of you (you shouldn't do it) . . . I think the main thing I worry about, is if and when the day comes that my kids find out the truth about me, if they're not adults then, it'll probably be a real disappointment to them, with their attitudes and the line of propaganda they've been fed, and I haven't really, you know I've never come out and said, you know I smoke pot and I'm proud of it, or I don't have a problem with it for myself, (my husband) and I talk about the Drug War, we talk about it in front of them, and how opposed we are to it. I don't think they've made the connection yet, why I might be opposed to it.

The changing risks she's witnessing during her marijuana use career are evident from the way she describes the time she got in trouble for her involvement with marijuana:

> The closest I came (to getting in trouble), one time I grew pot in the '70s and a policeman discovered it. But that was back in the 'good old days.' I just pulled it up (the marijuana plant she was growing in her yard) and gave it to him and he put it in a plastic sack. That was the end of that . . . it was *way* back then, I mean, it was kind of like a joke. I mean the cop was laughing . . . it was a funny story . . . today it wouldn't have had a very good ending.

When viewed in context of the large number of arrests for possession that occur today (Federal Bureau of Investigation [FBI], 2003), she is right. Leeza's case illustrates the on-going conflict and concern regarding detection faced by adult marijuana users, particularly those who live otherwise conventional lives. It is their involvement with marijuana, an illegal drug, which puts them at risk. The adults in this study have a lot to lose if their use is ever detected by those outside the small group of people who know about their marijuana use. Detection of use would almost inevitably lead to negative consequences in their lives. Users employed in professional occupations feared losing their jobs. Users with children feared having their children taken away. These adults are aware that even social (i.e., occasional) use is risky. In a society where there is no distinction between use and abuse, and no level of use is tolerated, the risks of being detected are real. This became clear during a discussion with Tom, a marijuana-using lawyer who stated that he would never have been willing to do an interview and discuss his marijuana use with anyone had he not been referred to the study by a close, trusted friend. His concerns are clearly valid.

For the majority of adult marijuana users, the activities related to acquiring and using marijuana were the only criminal activities they engaged in. They were not involved in other criminal or deviant behaviors. While maintaining access is a necessity for using marijuana (Becker, 1963), acquiring marijuana is illegal. Because of the intensified enforcement of marijuana offenses, growing marijuana is not an option for these users. Users purchase marijuana themselves, have others purchase it for them, or use it only when it is around. Andrea, a 36-year-old user, discussed how she got marijuana:

I have actually a couple of people . . . I mean I don't know how other users feel about this, but I like to be, you know there's sort of a chain you go through to get it, and I like to be down the chain. I don't like to be close to the actual source because I know where he's getting it. With another friend, not only is it safer, cheaper, and better quality, I don't know where he's getting it. And that is what I prefer, but again it just depends . . . it requires very little effort. It requires a phone call. It is incredibly easy to get. If I ask for it today, I could probably have it tonight. [Do you buy it yourself?] I don't purchase it directly from a dealer. I purchase it from a friend that purchases it from a dealer. I've never gotten it from a dealer. I don't want to do that.

It is clear her peers play an important role in helping her secure marijuana to use, thus minimizing the risks of having to purchase it from a dealer. Purchasing through her peer network reduces any risks associated with involvement in the black market. It is viewed as safer and reduces the likelihood of being detected or arrested. The fact that the majority of marijuana users were employed and were not engaged in other criminal activities is important to understanding how they afforded marijuana. The money they spent on marijuana came primarily from legitimate means. They talked about discontinuing their use or cutting down at times when they couldn't afford it. This was not a population of users who become involved in other criminal activities to support their marijuana use. Sean, for example, is a 52-year-old user who quit for a few years because he couldn't afford it:

I have (quit), um, when I got laid-off from my job . . . in 1992 and moved back to Oklahoma, I couldn't afford it, and I didn't buy any because I knew that I didn't want to spend any money on it, and for a year-and-a-half, I didn't smoke any marijuana, then I got a better job, got another job, so when I could afford it, then I started buying again and started smoking.

Only the few individuals who were engaged in dealing small amounts of marijuana to their peers were receiving some of their money from illegal means.

The context in which users consume marijuana also changes somewhat in adulthood. Use becomes integrated into activities that are suitable for marijuana use. Adult users discussed consuming marijuana while involved with other conventional activities, such as while watching TV, reading, or prior to playing golf with friends. This provides evidence that the users in this study are not immersed in a drug-using lifestyle, but rather use within the context of other conventional behaviors and activities. This is illustrated by Mark's description of a typical day that he might use marijuana:

> I will use it alone, but, I try to pick my spots, you know, um, you know, like again, if I have a day off, ____ (wife's) not here, I got no problem, you know, smoking some and doing the yard, you know 'cuz I love doing it, I love doing the yard and everything and it's just a, a nice, you know to me, it's a damn good day, it's just a damn good day to be able to be incredibly relaxed, walk around in sweat pants and, and aqua socks and do the, do the yard, yeah, you know just to live and to try to push all those things that we think are so fucking important all the time, out of there.

These contextual patterns applied even in situations where adult users were using marijuana with their peers. When adult users consumed with their peers, they remained involved in primarily conventional activities. Their activities were not limited to the consumption of marijuana, and marijuana use was not the central activity of group.

In addition to the reductions in illicit drug use among their peers, adult marijuana users become increasingly associated with peers and social contacts who do not use marijuana and who do not have knowledge of their use. Due primarily to its illegality, an individual's marijuana use can be a potential source of conflict between adult users and others who do not condone the use of an illegal drug. This is illustrated by Andrea's comments about how her peers handle knowledge of her marijuana use:

> [Who all knows about your marijuana use?] I would say that most everyone I know, knows. I don't, you know, the people I work with don't know, the people I worked with at my last job, some of them knew . . . and I think all of my friends know, although it isn't something that we talk about. I don't know how they really feel about it. I think some of them are completely accepting of it. I know one of my friends is *very* critical of it. We've talked about it a few times, you know, had a couple of heated conversations about it. No, she doesn't like it at all. She did that whole DARE thing and I think that she's just so full of propaganda that she can't see past

it. She's never used it. It makes a big difference, you know, I think she thinks that because it's illegal, it's bad.

To minimize the risks of being identified as a marijuana user, adult users restrict knowledge of their marijuana use, and use only in front of persons they trust intimately. Knowledge of their marijuana use is kept separate from most other social relationships. Sean's situation was common, in that only a few of the people in his life know about his marijuana use:

> My relatives don't know, um, but my (immediate) family does, my own family, my sisters and brothers know, um, my wife knows, um, all of my friends that smoke know, many of my friends that don't smoke know, but no one at work knows, and there's several other, some other people that I don't smoke marijuana in front of or let them know. Until someone's a good friend, I don't, and I know where they stand on the issue, I don't even (let them know I use) . . .

Particularly because the adult marijuana users in this study have a great deal to lose, they go to great lengths to keep their marijuana use separated from other parts of their lives. For the most part, they keep their use hidden and restrict knowledge of their use. In comparison to subcultures of users who are identifiable on the basis of their language, clothing or other characteristics, these users are difficult to detect. Because their lifestyles do not revolve around marijuana consumption, their involvement with marijuana use is not evident to most of the people in their lives. Only their close peers and certain family members are aware of their marijuana use.

## CONCLUSIONS

While the concept *maturation* (Winick, 1962) is typically used to refer to individuals who stop using illicit drugs in adulthood, there is evidence that by their own accounts, the adult marijuana users in this study have also experienced maturation. To the extent that they have passed through a phase of heavier illicit drug and through a period in which their lifestyles were more immersed in peer-related drug use, it can be stated that they have matured. To the extent that their patterns of marijuana use have changed as their life circumstances have changed, it can be said that they have matured. The majority of individuals in this study went through a phase of experimentation with illicit drugs in adolescence. Some used illicit substances only experimentally, while some developed more regular, sometimes problematic patterns of illicit drug use. Regardless, all experienced changes and reductions in their illicit drug use over time. By their own accounts, it is clear that their involvement with marijuana in adulthood differs in a number of ways from their patterns of use in adolescence. The social situations in which they use marijuana are now influenced by changes in use among their peers and changes in their lifestyles. As they become increasingly involved in maintaining their adult responsibilities, their views on marijuana change. It becomes of secondary importance to other life concerns. The users in this study are likely to differ in a number of ways from marijuana users who repeatedly come to the attention of the criminal justice system, and from problem users of the drug. The majority of them are legitimately employed and successful by most measures. They take care of their responsibilities, have families, and do not fit stereotypes about marijuana users. They minimize the risks of their marijuana involvement and keep their use from interfering in other aspects of their lives. Their consumption of marijuana is limited to their free time. The frequency of their use varies depending on other life factors. They constantly re-evaluate their use and alter the frequency of their use to fit into the conventional lifestyles they lead and want to maintain. They restrict knowledge of their marijuana involvement to a select group of close friends and family members who they can trust. These informal rules are similar to the social rituals and self-regulatory mechanisms that have been identified in other studies of controlled marijuana users (Cohen & Kaal, 2001; Zinberg et al., 1977). Marijuana use in this group did not impede individuals' abilities to maintain involvement in conventional roles and activities.

The adult marijuana users in this study view their marijuana use as a recreational, private activity, secondary to other roles and responsibilities. Their recreational use of marijuana is parallel to the notion of *time out*, identified among adolescent drug users in Britain (Parker et al., 1998). It is something they choose to do as a way to relax and take a break from life's stresses. For the adults in this study, marijuana consumption is not a central aspect of their self-identity or lifestyle. It is a recreational activity individuals engage in during their free time. Marijuana use is one of many activities individuals engage in during their leisure time. It is part of their self-identities to the extent that it is something they engage in, think about, and share in common with other users. However, it does not define who they are. Given the illegality of marijuana and risks thereof, adult users are cognizant that their involvement with marijuana makes them different from others. They keep knowledge of their use hidden from most of the people in their lives, and take steps to minimize the risks of being detected. Marijuana use is the only illegal behavior these adult users engage in. Even when marijuana is consumed among peers, it tends not to be the primary activity of the group. By their own accounts, these marijuana users make "rational" decisions about marijuana use. When making decisions about using marijuana, they think about the other things they have to do, how much leisure time they have, and who they are around. Adult marijuana users make choices about their marijuana involvement, and stop when they have other responsibilities to attend to. This serves as evidence of their control over their own marijuana use. Their recognition of the potential risks and consequences of their on-going marijuana involvement provides evidence that there is a cost-benefit assessment underlying their involvement with marijuana.

This study demonstrates the importance of taking variations among different types of drug users into account in drug research. The adult users in this study are likely to be different from problematic or compulsive users who are unable to control their use and function due to their involvement with marijuana. This is a population at risk for being labeled criminal on the basis of their recreational activity, a recreational activity that they are in control of. That the adult users in this study are able to control their drug use and limit the negative consequences of marijuana use on their lives coincides with arguments posited by others who have called for the issue of control to be incorporated into the discourse about illicit drug use (see Apsler, 1979; Zinberg, 1984; Zinberg & Harding, 1979). This is a perspective gaining attention with those who promote harm reduction (Inciardi & Harrison, 2000; Riley & O'Hare, 2000; Somers, Tapert, & Marlatt, 1992) and public health (Goldstein, 2001) approaches to drug policy.

## REFERENCES

Adler, Patricia A. (1993). *Wheeling and dealing: An ethnography of an upper-level drug dealing and smuggling community.* New York: Columbia University Press.
Apsler, Robert. (1979). Measuring how people control the amounts of substances they use. *Journal of Drug Issues, 9*(2), 145-159.

Babbie, Earl. (2005). *The basics of social research.* Belmont, CA: Thomson Wadsworth.

Bachman, Jerald G., Wadsworth, Katherine N., O'Malley, Patrick M., Johnston, Lloyd D., & Schulenberg, John E. (1997). *Smoking, drinking, & drug use in young adulthood.* Mahwah, NJ: Lawrence Erlbaum Associates.

Bachman, Jerald G., O'Malley, Patrick M., Schulenberg, John E., Johnston, Lloyd D., Bryant, Alison L., & Merline, Alicia C. (2002). *The decline of substance use in young adulthood.* Mahwah, NJ: Lawrence Erlbaum Associates.

Ball, John C., & Snarr, Richard W. (1969). A test of the maturation hypothesis with respect to opiate addiction. *Bulletin on Narcotics, 21*(4):9-13.

Becker, Howard S. (1953). Becoming a marihuana user. *American Journal of Sociology, 59,* 235-242.

Becker, Howard S. (1963). *Outsiders.* New York: The Free Press.

Biernacki, Patrick. (1986). *Pathways from heroin addiction.* Philadelphia: Temple University Press.

Biernacki, Patrick & Waldorf, D. (1981). Snowball sampling: Problems and techniques of chain referral sampling. *Sociological Methods & Research, 10,* 141-163.

Bourgois, Philippe. (2003). *In search of respect.* 2nd ed. New York: Cambridge University Press.

Brake, Mike. (1980). *The Sociology of youth culture and youth subcultures.* Boston: Routledge & Kegan Paul.

Canada, Parliament. (2003). *Cannabis: Report of the Senate Special Committee on Illegal Drugs.* Toronto, Canada: University of Toronto Press.

Charmaz, Kathy, & Mitchell, Richard G. (2001). Grounded theory in ethnography. In P. Atkinson, A. Coffey, S. Delamont & J. Lofland (Eds.), *Handbook of Ethnography* (pp. 160-174). Thousand Oaks: Sage Publications.

Chen, Kevin, & Kandel, Denise B. (1995). The natural history of drug use from adolescence to the mid-thirties in a general population sample. *American Journal of Public Health, 85*(1), 41-47.

Clarke, Ronald V., & Cornish, Derek B. (1985). Modeling offenders' decisions: A framework for research and policy. In M. Tonry & N. Morris (Eds.), *Crime & justice: An annual review of research* (Vol. 6) (pp. 147-185). Chicago: University of Chicago Press.

Clarke, Ronald V. & Cornish, Derek B. (2001). Rational choice. In R. Paternoster & Ronet Bachman (Eds.), *Explaining Criminals & Crime* (pp. 23-46). CA: Roxbury.

Cloward, Richard A. & Ohlin, Lloyd E. (1960). *Delinquency & opportunity.* New York: Free Press.

Cohen, Peter D.A., & Kaal, Hendrien L. (2001). *The irrelevance of drug policy: Patterns and careers of experienced cannabis use in the populations of Amsterdam, San Francisco and Bremen.* Amsterdam: CEDRO, University of Amsterdam.

Cornish, Derek B., & Clarke, Ronald V. (Eds.). (1986). *The reasoning criminal.* New York: Springer-Verlag.

Drug Enforcement Administration. 2003. *Illegal drug price & purity.* Drug Intelligence Report. April. Washington, DC: U.S. Department of Justice.

Earlywine, Mitch. (2002). *Understanding marijuana.* New York: Oxford University Press.

Federal Bureau of Investigation. (2003). *Crime in the United States 2002, Uniform Crime Reports.* Washington, DC: U.S. Department of Justice.

Glaser, Barney G., & Strauss, Anselm L. (1967). *The discovery of grounded theory: Strategies for qualitative research.* Chicago: Aldine Publishing Co.

Goldstein, Avram. (2001). *Addiction. 2nd* edition. NY: Oxford University Press.

Golub, Andrew, and Johnson, Bruce D. (1999). Cohort changes in illegal drug use among arrestees in Manhattan: From the heroin injection generation to the blunts generation. *Substance Use and Misuse, 34*(13), 1733-1763.

Golub, Andrew, and Johnson, Bruce D. (2001). *The rise of marijuana as the drug of choice among youthful adult arrestees.* (NCJ 187490). Washington, DC: National Institute of Justice.

Golub, Andrew, Johnson, Bruce, Dunlap, Eloise, & Sifaneck, Steve. (2004). Projecting and monitoring the life course of the Marijuana/Blunts Generation. *Journal of Drug Issues, 34*(2), 361-388.

Goode, Erich. (1970). *The marijuana smokers.* New York: Basic Books.

Hallstone, Michael. (2002). Updating Howard Becker's theory of using marijuana for pleasure. *Contemporary Drug Problems, 29*(4), 821-846.

Hirsch, Michael L., Conforti, Randell W., & Graney, Carolyn J. (1990). The use of marijuana for pleasure: A replication of Howard S. Becker's study of marijuana use. In J.W. Neuliep (Ed.), Handbook of Replication Research in the Behavioral and Social Sciences [Special Issue], *Journal of Social Behavior and Personality, 5*(4), 497-510.

Inciardi, James A., & Harrison, Lana D. (2000). Introduction. In J.A. Inciardi & L.D. Harrison (Eds.), *Harm Reduction* (pp. vii-xix). Thousand Oaks, CA: Sage.

Johnston, Lloyd D., O'Malley, Patrick M., & Bachman, Jerald G. (2001). *Monitoring the Future national survey results on drug use, 1975-2000. Secondary school students;* Vol. 1 (NIH publication 01-4924). *College students and adults ages 19-40.* (NIH publication 01-4925). Bethesda, MD: National Institute on Drug Abuse.

Johnston, Lloyd D., O'Malley, Patrick M., Bachman, Jerald G., & Schulenberg, John E. (2004). *Monitoring the Future national results on adolescent drug use: Overview of key findings, 2003.* (NIH Publication No. 04-5506). Bethesda, MD: National Institute on Drug Abuse.

Kandel, D.B., & Logan, J.A. (1984). Patterns of drug use from adolescence to young adulthood, I: Periods of risk for initiation, continued use and discontinuation. *American Journal of Public Health, 74,* 660-666.

Kandel, D.B., & Raveis, V.H. (1989). Cessation of Illicit Drug Use in Young Adulthood. *Arch Gen Psychiatry, 46,* 109-116.

Kandel, D.B., Yamaguchi, K., & Chen, K. (1992). Stages of progression in drug involvement from adolescence to adulthood: Further evidence for the gateway theory. *J. Stud. Alcohol, 53,* 447-457.

Labouvie, Erich (1996). Maturing out of substance use: Selection and self-correction. *Journal of Drug Issues, 26*(2):457-476.

Labouvie, Erich, & White, Helen R. 2002. Drug sequences, age of onset, and use trajectories as predictors of drug abuse/dependence in young adulthood. In D.B. Kandel (Ed.), *Stages and Pathways of Drug Involvement* (pp. 19-41). New York: Cambridge University Press.

Lindesmith, Alfred R. (1968). *Addiction and opiates.* Chicago: Aldine Publishing Co.

180      The Cultural/Subcultural Contexts of Marijuana Use

Mack, Alison, & Joy, Janet (2001). *Marijuana as Medicine?* Washington, DC: National Academy Press.

Maxwell, Joseph A. (1996). *Qualitative research design: An interactive approach.* (Applied Social Research Methods Series, Volume 41). Thousand Oaks: Sage.

McCambridge, John, & Strang, John (2004). Patterns of drug use in a sample of 200 young drug users in London. *Drugs: Education, prevention, and policy, 11*(2), 101-112.

Merline, Alicia C., O'Malley, Patrick M., Schulenberg, John E., Bachman, Jerald G., & Johnston, Lloyd D. (2004). Substance use among adults 35 years of age: Prevalence, adulthood predictors, and impact of adolescent substance use. *American Journal of Public Health, 94*(1), 96-102.

National Commission on Marihuana and Drug Abuse. (1972). *Marihuana: A signal of misunderstanding.* Washington, DC: U.S. Government Printing Office.

National Institute of Justice. (1999). *1998 annual report on marijuana use among arrestees.* (NCJ-175658). Washington, DC: National Institute of Justice.

National Institute of Justice. (2000). *Marijuana is drug of choice among Oklahoma City arrestees.* Office of Justice Programs News. Retrieved March 13, 2003, from http://www.adam-nij.net/files/release/oklahoma.pdf

National Institute of Justice. (2003). *2000 arrestee drug abuse monitoring: Annual report.* (NCJ 193013). U.S. Department of Justice: Washington, DC.

Neuman, Lawrence, & Weigand, Bruce. (2000). *Criminal justice research methods: Qualitative and quantitative approaches.* Needham Heights, MA: Allyn and Bacon.

Office of National Drug Control Policy. (2002). *Substance use in popular music videos.* Retrieved January 29, 2004 from http://www.whitehousedrugpolicy.gov

Office of National Drug Control Policy. (2004). *Marijuana.* Executive Office of the President. Retrieved July 15, 2004, from http://www.whitehousedrugpolicy.gov

Parker, Howard, Aldridge, Judith, & Measham, Fiona. (1998). *Illegal leisure.* New York: Routledge.

Riley, Diane, & O'Hare, Pat. (2000). Harm reduction: History, definition & practice. In J.A. Inciardi & L.D. Harrison (Eds.), *Harm Reduction* (pp. 1-26). Thousand Oaks: Sage.

SAMHSA. (2003). *Results from the 2002 national survey on drug use and health: National findings.* (Office of Applied Studies, NHSDA Series H-22, DHHS Publication No. SMA 03-3836). Rockville, MD: U.S. Department of Health and Human Services.

SAMHSA. (2004). *Results from the 2003 national survey on drug use and health: National findings.* (Office of Applied Studies, NSDUH Series H-25, DHHS Publication No. SMA 04-3964). Rockville, MD: U.S. Department of Health and Human Services.

Schwandt, Thomas A. (1997). *Qualitative inquiry.* Thousand Oaks: Sage.

Shukla, Rashi K. (2003). *A rational choice analysis of decision-making and desistance from marijuana use.* (Doctoral Dissertation, Rutgers University, 2003). *Dissertation Abstracts International, 64*, 1417.

Snow, M. (1973). Maturing out of narcotic addiction in New York City. *The International Journal of the Addictions, 8*(6):921-938.

Somers, Julian, Tarpert, Susan F., & Marlatt, G. Alan. (1992). Bringing harm reduction home. In A. Trebach & K.B. Zeese (Eds.), *Strategies for change: New directions for drug policy* (pp. 221-226). Washington DC: Drug Policy Foundation.

Stephens, Robert S. Roffman, Roger A., & Simpson, Edith E. (1993). Adult marijuana users seeking treatment. *Journal of Consulting & Clinical Psychology, 61*(6), 1100-1104.

Sterk, Claire E. (1999). *Fast lives: Women who use crack cocaine.* Philadelphia: Temple University Press.

Strauss, Anselm, & Corbin, Juliet. (1998). *Basics of qualitative research.* 2nd Ed. Thousand Oaks: Sage.

Sutter, Alan G. (1970). Worlds of drug use on the street scene. In J.H. McGrath & F.R. Scarpitti (Eds.), *Youth and Drugs* (pp. 74-86). Glenview, IL: Scott, Foresman, and Co.

Waldorf, Dan, Reinarman, Craig, & Murphy, Sheigla. (1991). *Cocaine changes.* Philadelphia: Temple University Press.

Warr, Mark. (1998). Life-course transitions & desistance from crime. *Criminology, 36*(2), 183-215.

Weiner, Michelle D., Sussman, Steve, McCullen, William J., & Lichtman, Kara. (1999). Factors in marijuana cessation among high-risk youth. *Journal of Drug Education, 29*(4), 337-357.

Williams, Terry. (1989). *The cocaine kids.* Cambridge, MA: Perseus Books.

Winick, Charles. (1962). Maturing out of narcotic addition. *Bulletin on Narcotics, 14:*1-7.

Zinberg, Norman E. (1984). *Drug, set and setting.* New Haven: Yale University Press.

Zinberg, Norman E., & Harding, Wayne M. (1979). Control & intoxicant use: A theoretical & practical overview. *Journal of Drug Issues, 9*(2), 121-143.

Zinberg, Norman E., Harding, Wayne M., & Winkeller, Miriam. (1977). A study of social regulatory mechanisms in controlled illicit drug users. *Journal of Drug Issues, 7*(2), 117-133.

# Mother's Milk and the Muffin Man: Grassroots Innovations in Medical Marijuana Delivery Systems

Wendy Chapkis, PhD
Richard J. Webb, PhD

**SUMMARY.** In the ongoing debates over medical marijuana, opponents often conflate the alleged risks of cannabis therapeutics with the acknowledged harms associated with smoking. Although smoking is the most widely used method of administering marijuana, it is not the only available means. This paper provides an account of the production, distribution, and administration of non-smokable cannabis products by members of a California health care collective, the Wo/Men's Alliance for Medical Marijuana. WAMM has developed a variety of alternative methods of administering cannabis orally and externally that challenge the rhetorical equivalence between smoking as a delivery method and botanical marijuana as a medicine. Their experience with low-cost and low-tech production techniques has enabled even the poor and uninsured among them to manage the debilitating symptoms of their illnesses and the side-effects of their often onerous courses of treatment, without smoking. The organization provides an informative example of

Wendy Chapkis is Associate Professor of Sociology and Women's Studies, University of Southern Maine (E-amil: chapkis@usm.maine.edu).

Richard J. Webb is Lecturer, Department of Communication Studies, San Jose State University.

[Haworth co-indexing entry note]: "Mother's Milk and the Muffin Man: Grassroots Innovations in Medical Marijuana Delivery Systems." Chapkis, Wendy, and Richard J. Webb. Co-published simultaneously in *Journal of Ethnicity in Substance Abuse* (The Haworth Press, Inc.) Vol. 4, No. 3/4, 2005, pp. 183-204; and: *The Cultural/Subcultural Contexts of Marijuana Use at the Turn of the Twenty-First Century* (ed: Andrew Golub) The Haworth Press, Inc., 2005, pp. 183-204. Single or multiple copies of this article are available for a fee from The Haworth Document Delivery Service [1-800-HAWORTH, 9:00 a.m. - 5:00 p.m. (EST). E-mail address: docdelivery@haworthpress.com].

Available online at http://www.haworthpress.com/web/JESA
doi:10.1300/J233v04n03_08

the way grassroots innovation and collective organization can challenge institutionalized assumptions about medicine, health care, and the alleviation of suffering. *[Article copies available for a fee from The Haworth Document Delivery Service: 1-800-HAWORTH. E-mail address: <docdelivery@ haworthpress.com> Website: <http://www.HaworthPress.com> © 2005 by The Haworth Press, Inc. All rights reserved.]*

**KEYWORDS.** Drug policy, medical marijuana, alternatives to smoking

## *INTRODUCTION*

Despite federal prohibitions on marijuana use, over the past decade several states have approved legislation that permits patients, under the care of a physician, to use cannabis for medicinal purposes. Federal opposition relies, in part, on concerns about the safety of a smoked botanical. Indeed, it is often an argument about the risks associated with smoking (the most widely used method of administering marijuana) that substitutes for the much weaker claims of the risks associated with cannabis itself.

Opponents of the medicinal use of marijuana side-step the fact that many alternative methods of administering the drug have been developed by grassroots groups and are available and in use. This article provides an account of the production, distribution, and administration of non-smokable cannabis products by members of a California health care collective, the Wo/Men's Alliance for Medical Marijuana (WAMM). After looking at the history of the regulation and prohibition of marijuana, and its justification by reference to the dangers of smoking, we discuss the wide range of alternatives produced at WAMM including baked goods, tinctures, capsules, soy-based beverages, and liniments. The production of these alternatives, and members' accounts of making and using them, reveal innovative strategies of harm-reduction and patient empowerment.

### *Cannabis Therapeutics*

Cannabis has a long history as a therapeutic substance, with the first recorded medicinal uses dating back more than two millennia (Grinspoon, 2000). In Western pharmacopoeias, it appeared a century and a half ago as "tincture of hemp" or "tincture of cannabis" and was readily available in the United States by prescription to treat a wide range of ailments until the passage of the 1937 Marijuana Tax Act (Grinspoon, 1994: 10). However, as synthetic analgesics became increasingly available, tinctures and other herbal remedies lost ground to medicines available as standardized pills (Grinspoon, 2000). Concerns about the recreational use of marijuana further undermined acceptance of cannabis as medicine and, in 1941, it was formally removed from the U.S. Pharmacopoeia and the National Formulary (Grinspoon, 1994: 218). With the passage of the Controlled Substances Act of 1970, marijuana was classified as a Schedule 1 drug, meaning it is considered unsafe even under medical supervision, with a high potential for abuse, and no accepted medical use.

Despite this discursive erasure of cannabis therapeutics, the medicinal use of marijuana continued. Indeed, six years after declaring marijuana without medicinal value, the federal government itself began providing marijuana to a small group of patients through the FDA's Investigational New Drug program (Randall, 1991; Zimmer and Morgan, 1997). Since 1996, eleven states have passed legislation endorsing the use of marijuana for medical purposes. Nonetheless, federal officials continue to steadfastly resist reclassification of marijuana to Schedule II or III under the Controlled Substances Act, which would permit patients to use it under the supervision of a physician. This resistance is ostensibly due to concerns about the lack of definitive evidence of either its safety or its efficacy. But researchers continue to face almost insurmountable hurdles in their attempts to receive federal approval to study the drug.[1] As a result, in 2000, there was only one clinical trial of the medical effects of cannabis underway in the United States, involving fewer than 70 volunteers (Guterman, 2000).

The scientific studies that have been done, however, suggest that concerns about the dangers of cannabis are exaggerated. In 1988, a DEA Administrative Law Judge, Francis Young, presided over hearings on the risks of marijuana use and concluded: "Marijuana in its natural form is one of the safest therapeutically active substances known" (Randall, 1989: 440). Similarly, Dr. Janet Joy, director of the 1999 Institute of Medicine report on "Marijuana and Medicine: Assessing the Science Base," has argued that concerns about the physiological effects of cannabis on the immune system have not been well established and the possibility that users could become dependent on the drug is "well within the risks we already tolerate [with other medicines]" (Guterman, 2000: 4).

The only clearly established adverse effect of sustained marijuana use is associated, not with the plant itself, but with one of its most common delivery systems: smoking. Researchers studying the effects of chronic marijuana smoking have concluded that lung function is impaired in much the same way as with heavy tobacco smoking; indeed, "marijuana smoke and tobacco smoke are rather similar. Many of the toxic compounds, such as tar, carbon monoxide, and cyanide, are found in comparable levels in both types of smoke" (Kuhn et al., 2003: p. 144). The 1999 Institute of Medicine report on marijuana as medicine notes that "numerous studies suggest that marijuana smoke is an important risk factor in the development of respiratory disease" (ES-6). The IOM report is clear, however, that it is smoking–not the use of the plant itself–that is of concern: ". . . except for the harms associated with smoking, the adverse effects of marijuana use are within the range tolerated for other medicines" (3.49). Indeed, the IOM report strongly recommends research into alternative delivery systems for a substance that appears to be so therapeutically promising: "The argument against the future of smoked marijuana for treating any condition is not that there is no reason to predict efficacy, but that there is risk. That risk could be overcome by the development of a non-smoked, rapid-onset delivery system for cannabinoid drugs" (4.42).

But because smoking is well established as hazardous, while marijuana itself is not, opponents of the legalization of even the medicinal uses of cannabis frequently focus on the dangers of the delivery system as a stand-in for missing or weak arguments about the dangers of the botanical drug itself. At an April 2004 Congressional hearing on medical marijuana, the chair of the subcommittee–and an outspoken opponent of marijuana use–Representative Mark Souder (R-IN)–used the IOM report to dismiss the possibility that the botanical form of the drug might have any medicinal value. To establish this point, he noted that the IOM report "stressed that smoking marijuana is not safe, not a safe medical delivery device, and exposes patients to a significant number of harmful substances" (hearing transcript: 3).

Repeatedly during the hearings, risks of smoking are raised as the reason why whole-plant, botanical cannabis should not be considered an appropriate medicinal substance. Dr. Robert Meyer, Director of the FDA's Office of Drug Evaluation, in his testimony before the committee, for example, observed that while some components within cannabis appear to be therapeutically active, "Marijuana, botanical marijuana, is not an approved drug" (hearing transcript: 3). Souder immediately followed this observation with the suggestion that any cannabinoid medication would be distinct from the botanical plant: "And it wouldn't be marijuana? It would be some component inside the marijuana." Meyer's response is telling: "Well, again, I think there are inherent toxicities to smoking anything" (hearing transcript: 5). The substance in its botanical form becomes synonymous with the delivery system of smoking. At the end of his testimony, Meyer returned to the question of herbal or botanical medicine, arguing that "FDA does not have an inherent bias against botanical products. If botanical products are developed correctly and shown to be safe and effective . . . we would approve of a botanical product" (hearing transcript: 7). Souder immediately interjected, "Do you have any smoked products you've approved?" Meyer replied, "I don't believe so. No" (hearing transcript: 7). Once again, the botanical form of the drug is reduced to a "smoked product."

This rhetorical strategy has been deployed in more popular venues as well. A July 2004 Fox television program, the O'Reilly Factor, featured an interview with Dr. Andrea Barthwell, the U.S. Deputy Drug Czar. O'Reilly asked his guest if she wouldn't agree with him that certain seriously ill individuals–such as TV celebrity Montel Williams, living with MS–should have access to doctor-recommended marijuana. O'Reilly: "If a doctor–*a doctor*–says that he needs it for his MS, he should have it. You don't disagree with that, do you?" Barthwell: "Well, I do, actually. There is nothing that tells us from the science now that smoked, crude botanical should be a medication" (transcript of O'Reilly Factor 2004).

One notable exception to this approach among prominent public health officials has been articulated by former U.S. Surgeon General Joycelyn Elders. In a published editorial in the spring of 2004, Dr. Elders observed that "Marijuana does not need to be smoked. Some patients prefer to eat it, while those who need the fast action and dose control provided by inhalation can avoid the hazards of smoke through simple devices called vaporizers" (Elders, 2004). Her acknowledgment of alternative delivery systems presents a clear challenge to those within the federal bureaucracy who oppose the medicinal uses of the plant on the basis of the risks of smoking.

But rather than seriously exploring the medicinal uses of marijuana, most public officials at the federal level continue to challenge cannabis as a "smoked botanical." This narrow focus is justified by the claim that medical marijuana users and supporters are just druggies defending their access to joints. Dr. Robert Dupont (the first Director of the National Institute on Drug Abuse), for example, argued in his testimony to the Congressional sub-committee in 2004: "Much of the [legitimate] talk about medical marijuana is dealing with individual chemicals in it and not with the smoked marijuana . . .[But] the smoked marijuana is the only way it's interesting to the advocates in the field. They show no interest in the development of individual chemicals whatsoever. And that shows that their purpose is not medical. It's a way of influencing the country's policies toward marijuana. The legitimization of smoking marijuana, you can see that very clearly, with how little interest they have in individual chemicals or any delivery system, any delivery system other than smoking. They're only interested in smoking" (hearing transcript: 10).

Dupont's claims, however, are not supported by the evidence. Indeed, efforts by members of grassroots medical marijuana organizations, such as the Wo/Men's Alliance for Medical Marijuana, to create and to use non-smoked forms of cannabis-based medicines suggest that what these organizations oppose is not alternative delivery systems but corporate control of health care.

### What Is WAMM?

The Wo/Men's Alliance for Medical Marijuana was founded in Santa Cruz, California, in 1996 by medical marijuana patient Valerie Corral and her husband, Michael.[2] In April 2004, WAMM drew national and international attention when it won a temporary injunction against the U.S. Justice Department in federal district court; as a result, the organization was able to operate the only legally protected medical marijuana garden in the United States until the injunction was lifted in 2005 following the U.S. Supreme Court ruling in the Raich case.[3] WAMM is organized as a cooperative, composed primarily of low-income patients living with life-threatening illnesses. There are roughly 200 current members using medical marijuana, and another 70 supporting members serving as primary caregivers. Together they cultivate marijuana plants and produce a variety of medicinal products, which are made available to the membership according to need and without charge.[4] Instead of paying for their marijuana, members are encouraged, as their health permits, to contribute volunteer hours to the organization by working in the garden, assisting with fund raising, making cannabis tinctures, beverages, capsules, and baked goods, helping each other with informal hospice care, or volunteering in the office. Inevitably, some members become too ill to contribute, but their weekly medicine continues to be provided by those who are healthy enough to shoulder the burden. The sickest members, those who can do the least for the collective, are generally those whose need is also greatest.

The WAMM members interviewed for this project reported use of marijuana with a physician's recommendation for a range of conditions including nausea related to chemotherapy (for cancer and AIDS), spasticity (MS), seizures (epilepsy), and chronic and acute pain. In order to become members of WAMM, each of the patient participants discussed with their doctors the possible therapeutic value of marijuana and were told explicitly (and in writing) that cannabis might prove useful in managing the specific symptoms associated with their illness, disability, or course of treatment. The number of members the program can accommodate is limited by the amount of marijuana the organization is able to grow. There is an extensive waiting list to join the organization; with more than 80% of members living with a life-threatening illness, the standing joke is that "people are literally dying to get into WAMM."[5]

Financial support for the organization comes largely from external donations. In 1998, however, the federal government revoked WAMM's non-profit status on the grounds that it was involved in supplying a federally prohibited substance. WAMM's struggle for survival further intensified in the fall of 2002, when the federal Drug Enforcement Administration raided the WAMM garden, eradicated a year's supply of medical marijuana, and arrested the two co-founders (however, to date, no charges have been filed against them). Despite these challenges, WAMM has continued to operate with the full support of California elected officials and in close cooperation with local law enforcement agencies. On April 21, 2004, Judge Jeremy Fogel of the federal district court in San Jose, citing the Ninth Circuit Court of Appeals' decision in *Raich v. Ashcroft*, barred the U.S. Attorney General and the Drug Enforcement Administration from interfering with the Corrals, WAMM patients, or the collective's garden. The federal injunction provided at least temporary respite in the ongoing battle with the federal government. Over the past decade, WAMM has operated as both a social experiment in community health care and a grassroots research project on the delivery and efficacy of multiple forms of medical marijuana.

## *METHOD*

This paper is part of a book length research project (*Dying to Get High*, New York University Press, forthcoming) on WAMM and the politics of medical marijuana use and provision. Our research is not intended as an investigation into whether cannabis is, in fact, an effective or appropriate medicine. Rather it is a richly detailed ethnographic account of the role of cannabis and community in the lives of one group of medical marijuana users and their struggle to secure the right to collectively produce and to use this "herbal medicine."

As researchers, we did not enter the field as dispassionate observers. We came to the subject of medical marijuana believing that doctors should have the right to recommend non-toxic herbs to their patients in an effort to relieve suffering, and that patients should have the right to obtain and to use such substances. Our status as sympathetic, though not uncritical, allies was fundamental to our ability to gain access to this community. WAMM is, after all, an organization under siege, and its members have every reason to be concerned about the motives of outsiders.

Data collection began in 1998 and is ongoing. Research has involved not only attendance at weekly membership meetings during which medical marijuana is provided to member patients, but also included volunteer work in the collective's garden and participation in a variety of organizational activities. Open-ended interviews were conducted with three dozen WAMM members. Most interview subjects came forward voluntarily from the general WAMM membership; these initial interviews were supplemented with key person interviews (including interviews with the co-founders of the organization, several members of the board of directors, and local law enforcement and elected officials). Targeted interviewing within WAMM was also employed to ensure that the interview sample reflected the diversity within the membership (including differences of race, class, gender, sexual orientation, and physical condition). In addition to this primary research, we also engaged in an extensive review of relevant drug and health policy literature, and assembled an archive of newspaper reports, articles, and photographs related to WAMM and to legal battles over medical marijuana. From the outset we were explicit about our commitment to establishing a relationship with our informants that acknowledged their interests and expertise, and that is consistent with the overriding organizational values of WAMM: compassion and empowerment.

All of our informants are legal medical marijuana users protected under California Health and Safety Code Sec. 11362. However, because of continuing federal prohibitions, interview subjects were encouraged to remain anonymous unless they specifically (and in writing) requested to be known by name. Our initial assumption was that most of those who would select to be publicly identified would be high profile activists or public officials. Significantly, however, many "ordinary" WAMM members demanded to be "known subjects." Pamela Cutler, for example, a young woman living with metastatic breast cancer, explained, "This is *my* story, my legacy. Use my name." The question of "legacy" has a particular resonance for the very seriously ill members of WAMM; many of the individuals whose accounts shape this project, including Pamela Cutler, have since died. For those individuals who requested anonymity, names and identifying information have been changed. In this paper, anonymous subjects are identified by a first-name-only pseudonym, while intentionally self-identifying subjects are referenced by both first and last names.

Our findings, of course, are based upon a single and somewhat unique organization, one that has achieved an unusual degree of influence within the medical marijuana movement. WAMM also operates within a civic community that is perhaps unusually supportive of medical marijuana users; consequently, our findings may not be readily generalizable across broader social and political contexts. Nor can we claim to provide a comprehensive analysis of members' perspectives, since only those who volunteered were interviewed; a small number of members were unwilling to participate due to lingering fears of federal prosecution, should their identities be compromised. Despite these limitations, this case study provides an important illustration of the ways that terminally ill and chronically suffering patients can benefit from cannabis therapeutics and collective organization.

## FINDINGS

### Smoking May Be Hazardous to Your Health

Interviews with WAMM members reveal that most have thought seriously about the possible risks of smoking as a delivery system and that many have attempted to reduce (or, in some cases, to eliminate) their reliance on smoking in favor of consuming baked goods, tinctures, or beverages, or using a vaporizer. However, for some–especially those living in the final stages of terminal illness–the benefits of smoked marijuana may, in fact, outweigh any long-term risks. Indeed, the IOM report acknowledges that this is to be expected: "it will likely be many years before a safe and effective cannabinoid delivery system, such as an inhaler, will be available for patients. In the meantime, there are patients with debilitating symptoms for whom smoked marijuana might provide relief . . . Because of the health risks associated with smoking, smoked marijuana should generally not be recommended for long-term medical use. Nonetheless, for certain patients, such as the terminally ill or those with debilitating symptoms, the long-term risks are not of great concern" (ES 8).

"Jon," who is living with AIDS, observes:

> I for one don't have a major concern about smoking. I feel like I'm already dealing with everything knick-knack-paddy-whack that could kill you. This disease is probably going to kill me eventually. So if the worst is that I have some side-effects because of smoking, oh well. Oh fucking well. And that's where I'm at with it. Because the side-effects of my meds are going to eventually take my organs. So if the marijuana smoke takes my lungs, so be it. But not everyone in our collective feels that way. Not everyone can smoke. So they use the baked goods. And when I don't want to smoke, I do eat the muffins instead of having to fire up.

Indeed, for many WAMM members, especially those living with chronic conditions or in remission from life-threatening illnesses, smoking is a serious concern. "Mary," a woman in her forties who uses cannabis for relief from the effects of breast cancer treatment, observes:

> I use pot by smoking it simply because I have yet to find another route where I get the same sort of effect. But it is a major concern of mine. My sister died about a year ago of lung cancer. Of course, she smoked a phenomenal amount of tobacco; she smoked like three packs a day for thirty years. I don't fall in that category with my pot; my god. But even still, it's smoking. And ever since she's died, every single time I smoke, a little light in the back of my head goes off reminding me that that's not great. I mean, it's great now, and I weigh the benefit versus risk, and the benefit definitely outweighs the risks for me–especially considering how little I consume compared to a cigarette smoker. But still, if I can find another route that will give me the same degree of relief, I'd switch in a heart beat. It's something I'm very conscious of. It's like right there in front of me.

Susan Durst, a 62-year-old woman with both personal and family experience of cancer, has similar concerns about smoking:

I have two parents who died of primary lung cancer and my lungs are a big concern to me. I've had breast cancer and so many of my friends have had their cancers metastasize to their lungs. So of course I worry about lung cancer. Instead of smoking, I tend to just eat a little bit of a [cannabis infused] muffin.

Some members who need the rapid onset properties of inhaled cannabis reduce the need to smoke by using a vaporizer which heats, but does not burn, the plant material. "James," a WAMM member who uses marijuana to offset the side-effects of AIDS medications, shifted from smoking to a vaporizer:

I know there is probably some damage to the lungs from smoking marijuana. After all, smoking is not a normal thing for humans to do, you know, to intake smoke. So we use a vaporizer, a "huffer," where we don't take in smoke. It's just fumes basically. But it's so potent. I get into coughing fits if it's full of fresh bud. My partner [also a WAMM member living with AIDS] can smoke the green, but I have to wait until after the initial burning. He uses it first, and then I can smoke what we call the second burning. Otherwise I get a cough like no other cough I've had in my life. I mean lights go on, things get sparkly. I don't know what burns off in that first burning. I mean, it's not even really burning. There is no fire involved. But whatever it is, I can't handle it if it's full of fresh bud.

As James' account suggests, the vaporizer works well for some individuals, less well for others. In addition to the variable physical effects of inhaling fumes produced by the vaporizer, some individuals find the machine itself to be off-putting. "David," 43 and living with AIDS, turned to a vaporizer as an alternative to smoking "spliffs" (tobacco mixed with marijuana) but notes:

I bought a vaporizer, but it's huge. It's like a chemistry set. I can't stand the thing so I just haven't put it to use.

## WAMM and Alternatives to Smoking

For members who do not need the rapid onset of inhaled cannabis, a range of other alternatives is produced by the collective, including baked goods, a soymilk-based beverage, and tinctures. This is both a response to the needs of members who cannot or choose not to smoke, and a reflection of the fact that the collective's garden produces a significant quantity of leaf matter in addition to the buds used for smoking or vaporizing. Both the leaves (which are removed periodically throughout the growing season to increase sunlight to the buds) and the more potent buds themselves contain the therapeutically active properties of the plant. James observes that, after the Drug Enforcement Administration raid on the collective's garden in 2002, the organization had to reduce the amount of bud provided to the members in order to make the previous year's supply stretch. This meant that members were encouraged to try the other products made of the more abundant leaf matter:

> I pulled way back on my smoking after the bust. We thought we had better hold on to what we had so I upped my eating because we had a lot of leaf. And I discovered that eating it has a different effect. It has an amazing effect on [pain from neuropathy in] my feet and legs.

James' observation that eating cannabis-based products has a different effect than smoking was widely reported by members. One 54-year-old woman with MS explained that the effectiveness of cannabis in relieving her symptoms depends entirely on the delivery system:

> My doctor who is treating me for the MS asked me if I would be interested in trying marijuana to see if I would get relief. He didn't want me to smoke it, though, because of lung damage. I wasn't interested in smoking it either because I knew from past experience that it didn't work; I only hurt afterwards when I smoked it. But I had never tried eating it for that purpose. When I did try it for the pain and had the opportunity to eat the leaf, I was really pleased. It really worked.

"Cher," a 52-year-old with a seizure disorder, helped to develop one of WAMM's alternative delivery methods, "Mother's Milk," because she found that smoking wasn't effective in treating her condition:

> My seizures were controlled with medications of all different sorts for a very long time but I kept complaining to my doctor about the side effects of the pharmaceuticals. Then he tried me on Marinol[6] because he thought it would have fewer side effects. But after two months, my insurance company said they would no longer cover it. And smoking [marijuana] wasn't enough to stop the seizures; it

wasn't the same as Marinol. So that's how I figured out about the milk. I think I kind of invented it. I would boil the bud in milk and drink it. And I could use the same bud maybe four or five times. I started with regular milk, but that upset my stomach so I switched to soy. Even the soy milk upsets my stomach a little, but it works. On 'Mother's Milk,' I feel better than I had on drugs and better than I had on Marinol.

While non-smoked forms of cannabis work well for many patients, one common concern is the challenge of establishing appropriate dosage. Patients report that unlike smoking, where they can easily control how much they ingest, eating cannabis-based products requires some experimentation to establish an effective–but not overpowering–dose. "Codi," a 49-year-old woman with glaucoma-related blindness and pain, explains:

I like to smoke it the most because I have more control over what I'm doing, of the level. If I've done a pipeful, I know what I've done. If I've rolled a cigarette, I know what I'm getting. But when I'm away from the house, I feel like I have to be very, very careful that there's no odor or anything from smoking so I'll use the muffins or the brownies if I'm going somewhere. I'll use a half a brownie, a fourth of a brownie. I don't want to be too medicated; I just want to take away the pain. That's it because with loss of vision, you already have so many other things to deal with. I actually like the soy milk a lot because you can freeze a little in those ice cube trays. Sometimes if I'm not feeling well, my daughter will make me a cup of tea and put a cube in. But I still feel that, with smoking, I have more control.

Both eating and smoking cannabis for therapeutic purposes requires a process of learning how to consume the plant-based medicine and how to recognize an effective dose.[7] "Jon," a 37-year-old with HIV, describes the process he went through learning how to both smoke and to eat medicinal marijuana:

I wasn't a smoker, so I knew that if I was going to smoke marijuana, I would have to get used to it. Instead I thought maybe if I would just ingest it, it would be easier for me. And it was easier but generally the effects either lasted way longer than I wanted or it took too long a time for me to get the effect. When I had my first muffin, I think I ate the whole thing. Within an hour or two I was so over the rainbow, I didn't know where I was. It was a really wonderful eye-opener. So then I started halving my muffins, if I took muffins. But often times, I needed something more immediate. The transition between doing muffins and smoking was a huge thing because, as I said, I just wasn't used to smoking. I had to learn how to do it . . . It was all a little trial and tribulation at first, learning how to smoke and learning how to ingest.

The development by WAMM members of alternative methods of ingestion has also been a learning, and teaching, process. As a grassroots collective, members were necessarily involved in, and in control of, each step of the complex and labor-intensive process of developing new drug delivery systems and learning how to use them. In the next section, we offer examples of the labor of love through which patients invented, and improved on, the organizations' many non-smoked medical marijuana products.

### Grassroots Innovations

On Saturday mornings in January, as the coastal fog rises above the Santa Cruz Mountains, eight WAMM members arrive at the collective's marijuana garden site for some volunteer labor. The two-hundred plants which grew there the summer before have been harvested and dried. The flowering tops, or "buds," have been trimmed and vacuum sealed in plastic bags. The buds are reserved for smoking, but every other part of the plant is utilized in non-smokable alternatives. The members are here to process the leaves, stems, and trimmings into the active ingredients of a variety of alternative cannabis products.

During the harvest and cleaning processes, primary attention is, of course, devoted to the buds, which are the most potent part of the plant. The bud trimmings, however, are collected and stored in small kitchen garbage bags, and the leaves are dried and stored in black plastic trash bags. The stems are saved, too, and set aside for the production of liniment.

In an effort to provide consistency in dosage, the bags of leaf are mixed together in barrels, evening out most of the variations in potency that may occur between plants. The leaf is then ground into powder using electric blenders. "You must remove the stems," cautions one volunteer, "or they will kill your blender." Grinding takes quite a while–only a handful or two can be ground at a time, and it can take half an hour or more before that much leaf is sufficiently pulverized. The blenders whine for hours, day after day, as the volunteers, most wearing earplugs, work their way through the mountain of marijuana leaves. Despite the conscientious removal of the stems, the blender attrition rate is shocking, and WAMM members continually scour the flea markets and resale shops looking for replacements.

The ground leaf is then spread onto an extremely fine-mesh screen suspended in a wooden framework above a shallow, rectangular wooden box. A glass plate lines the bottom of the box, and when the leaf powder is rubbed vigorously over the surface of the screen, the finest cannabis flour, called *kif*, falls through the mesh and is collected on the surface of the glass. The flour-like *kif* is used in the production of baked goods, and the coarser powder that remains on top of the screen is used to make marijuana capsules, tinctures and beverages.[8] Anything left over, material that would ordinarily be considered waste, is combined with the stems in producing cannabis liniment, used externally for the treatment of muscle and joint pain.

### Muffin Man

Until his death in 2003, "Johnny" was the Muffin Man. His baking routine began on Monday afternoon, with preparation of the dried cannabis leaf he would use to produce his marijuana muffins. Johnny preferred to process the leaf he used at home by himself, grinding it first in a blender, then running it through a coffee grinder in order to produce a flour that would not be grainy once baked. The leaf powder was then stirred into an ancient electric crock pot containing melted butter, vegetable oil, and water, where it would slowly cook on the lowest possible setting for the next 24 hours. Johnny firmly believed that the longer the leaf powder was allowed to cook, the more potent the resulting muffins would be, and it was to this practice that he attributed his success whenever patients mentioned their uncommon effectiveness. By Tuesday afternoon, the mixture in the crock pot was a dark green custard, of a consistency that Johnny was very particular about. The cooked leaf mixture was then blended with commercial chocolate cake mix and a few eggs, poured into muffin tins, and shoved into the oven to bake. Once Johnny had things rolling, there might be two dozen muffins in the oven, another three dozen cooling beside the window, and he would be dropping colorful paper cupcake liners into the next set of pans ready to be filled with batter. Wire racks covered with muffins sat on the countertop beside the sink, waiting until they were cool enough to be bagged. This, too, he was very particular about, and Johnny often missed the beginning of a Tuesday evening WAMM meeting because he had to wait a little longer for the muffins to cool.

Johnny rarely used his muffins for medicinal purposes, being inclined by preference and the nature of his illness toward smoking marijuana instead of eating it. But he found pleasure and purpose in the weekly ritual of baking for others and in being able to provide marijuana in a form that members who could not or who chose not to smoke would still be able to access. He was also just a bit perversely proud of the fact that new members were warned by old timers to approach the muffins with caution. They were generally so strong that many regular users recommended eating only a half, or even a quarter, of a muffin at a time. A few members found them unpleasantly strong and resorted to other alternatives, and several claimed that a whole muffin would put them to sleep for hours, although whether this was reported as a desirable effect or an undesirable one varied between patients.

### Mother's Milk

"Dianne" is fond of telling the story about her first experience with "Mother's Milk," a soy and cannabis beverage that was recommended to her for relief from chronic back pain. She consumed a bit more than might have been strictly necessary, and found not only pain relief, but almost forgotten feelings of sensuality and, afterward, a long, deep, restful sleep. "It's a body high, not a head high–very relaxing," she reports. She professes to exercise greater moderation since that day, but she remains particularly committed to the production and use of Mother's Milk.

For several years, a team of volunteers produced gallons of Mother's Milk every week, but members were unreliable about returning the reusable glass bottles in which it was distributed, and it became too costly for the organization to continue to replace them. Only a few members now go to the trouble of producing their own, but Dianne is among them. She receives an ounce of ground leaf powder each week. She pours the leaf powder, along with two quarts of soy milk and two quarts of water, into a large crock pot. She often adds a cinnamon stick for flavor, then cooks the mixture on the lowest possible heat for thirteen hours. Her husband then helps her strain the cooked milk though a fine-mesh tea strainer, then through a gold coffee filter–twice. The pale green beverage that remains is bottled and refrigerated. Dianne consumes about six ounces of Mother's Milk with her dinner, and that "takes care of me for the evening." She complains that occasionally it upsets her stomach, but it always provides rapid relief from her pain, muscle spasms, and paresthesia.

## Capsules

Organic, whole-plant, medical marijuana comes in pill form as well. Cannabis capsules, known as "Mari-caps," are produced twice a month by a six-person team of "Happy Cappers," led by long-time WAMM member, "Jon."

The whole team works together separating by hand the 1,200 gelatin capsules that will be filled with a mixture of ground leaf and butter. This mixture is cooked in quantity beforehand, very slowly at low temperature, and then frozen. While the capsules are being separated, the mixture is thawed until it becomes sufficiently pliable, although Jon reports that "sometimes, when there is too much butter in the blend, it gets pretty sticky, and it slows you down. It works better when it's stiffer, more granular."

Once separated, the bottom half of each capsule is inserted into a plastic tray–like a tiny ice cube tray–that holds fifty of them securely, their openings flush with its surface. A large, soft, dollop of cannabis mixture is pressed into the capsules by scraping it across the surface of the tray, using spoons or plastic cards. The mixture is then tamped into each capsule with a special tool that allows all fifty capsules to be firmly packed at once. Before purchasing the tamper, the crew packed each capsule, one at a time, using the end of a chopstick. At least three pressings and tampings are required before the capsules are completely filled, then the tops are placed on the capsules and all of them are wiped clean of any residue before being packaged. The capsules are packaged seven to twenty-eight per bag, for patients who use from one to four of them per day.

The effect is reportedly much like what is experienced from eating part of one of Johnny's muffins, with a delay of thirty minutes to an hour-and-a-half before the effects are noticeable, and a duration much longer than is customary with smoked marijuana, from four to eight, ten, or even twelve hours, according to some patients. Also like muffins, the capsules can be a bit unpredictable due to variations in potency, a problem that is being addressed by mixing the leaves of all the plants together before processing, in the hope that a consistent final product will result. The capsules are good, Jon says, because sometimes "downing a pill is easier than consuming a whole muffin, even though the pills can be a little tough on the stomach, sometimes, too." The capsules provide patients who are unable to smoke, either due to respiratory difficulties or social contexts in which smoking might be inappropriate, with an entirely unobtrusive alternative.

### Tincture

"Charlene" holds up a canning jar filled with an opaque, greenish-black liquid: cannabis tincture, the mildest (i.e., least psychoactive) of the orally administered non-smokables. She removes the lid and, holding it beneath a lamp, points to a surface that appears slightly reddish with iridescent flecks of a rusty golden hue. The THC extract floats to the top, she explains, and because of its tint is called "dragon's blood."

Producing the tincture is simple, Charlene explains, "easier than making pickles." Fill a canning jar about three-quarters of the way with ground cannabis leaf. Pour 151-proof alcohol over the cannabis, filling the jar almost to the top, but leaving just a little room so that it can be stirred and shaken. Cap the jar tightly, and store it in a warm, dark place for at least two weeks, longer if possible. The jar should be shaken at least a couple of times a week–preferably once or twice a day–to keep the ground cannabis in suspension and prevent sedimentation.

Once the ground leaf has steeped in alcohol for a sufficient time, Charlene's caregiver helps her decant the mixture, pouring it through a metal tea strainer or a piece of cheesecloth into a Pyrex beaker. Then, using a small glass funnel, Charlene fills the small bottles that will be distributed to patients. She delivers twenty 1-oz. bottles, four 2-oz. bottles, and one 4-oz.bottle of tincture a week. (The four ounce bottle is used by a multiple sclerosis patient with severe spasticity. One patient, a brittle diabetic, used 20 ounces a week; he reported that it got him off methadone.)

Cleanup is perhaps the most labor intensive part of the process. Charlene is comically emphatic about the superiority of one particular dishsoap, claiming that it outperforms all the others when it comes to dissolving THC residue. After washing, the jars and bottles are sterilized by boiling the glass parts and soaking the droppers in a diluted chlorine bleach bath, and then giving them a triple rinse.

The effect is different from that accompanying smoking, and also from that produced by baked goods, capsules, or mother's milk: the tincture has a mild sedative effect, rather than a pronounced "high." Charlene reports that, "One member used it for nausea at work, because she couldn't be high at work, and the tincture helped her without impairing her on the job. It's also ideal for nerve pain, and for muscle spasticity in patients with MS [multiple sclerosis], Parkinson's disease, and post-polio [syndrome]. It works immediately. It stops my muscle spasms, and reduces the nerve pain and hypersensitivity." Her pain and hypersensitivity are worst at night, she explains, and a cup of tea with the recommended dose of three teaspoons (three eye-droppers full) of tincture is enough to settle her for the night.

Like the other non-smokables, tincture is easy to use in public, when traveling or visiting, or when respiratory ailments make smoking uncomfortable or unadvisable. Because of its minimal psychoactive effect, it is often recommended to new members who have no history of marijuana use or who dislike the "high" that often accompanies the other medicinal products. It works rapidly and, like smoking, the patient can titrate–using just a little, pausing to gauge the effect, and tailoring the dose to his or her immediate requirements. Charlene also notes that any patient can make his or her own medicine, providing an empowering sense of self-control over one's symptoms.

### Liniment

"Tasha" is petite and grandmotherly, with curly gray hair and bifocals. She smiles broadly and her eyes light up when talking about the cannabis liniment she produces, a balm known among WAMM members as "rub-a-dub."

At the end of the medicinal marijuana production line, after the *kif* has been given to the bakers and the ground leaf has been used to produce tincture, capsules, and Mother's Milk, pounds and pounds of stems and leaf fragments remain. These former waste products, residue from the harvest and cleaning processes, were once tossed onto the mulch pile, until Tasha, who suffers from debilitating rheumatoid arthritis, revived the ancient practice of using cannabis in an alcohol solution as a poultice for her swollen, painful joints. For two years now, Tasha has produced rub-a-dub for any WAMM member who desires it.

The process is the simplest of all. Tasha scoops "a couple of pounds" of stems and leaves into a five-gallon jar, fills the jar to the top with rubbing alcohol, covers it, and stores it in a dark corner of her garage. After a month or more has gone by, she pours the dark green solution through a filter screen and back into the original rubbing alcohol bottles.

Tasha sometimes puts the rub-a-dub into a small spray bottle, or moistens a washcloth with it and applies it directly to her painful joints. She reports complete and rapid pain relief, lasting for about an hour.

Tasha recently discovered a five-gallon jar of rub-a-dub that had been hidden away in a corner of the garage and overlooked for a year. Its analgesic effects were considerably more powerful, she reports, her eyebrows arching in enthusiasm. Although demand for rub-a-dub normally forces her turn each batch over after only a month or so, she admitted that she has a couple of long-term batches secreted away.

## CONCLUSION

Over the past decade, the members of WAMM have developed a variety of alternative methods of administering cannabis orally and externally that challenge the rhetorical equivalence between smoking as a delivery method and botanical marijuana as a medicine. Their experience with low-cost and low-tech production techniques has enabled even the poor and uninsured among them to access a physician-recommended herbal medicine in an effort to manage debilitating symptoms of their illnesses and the side-effects of their often onerous courses of treatment. One result of their medical marijuana use and their membership in WAMM has been an increased sense of patient empowerment as the members successfully produce their own medication and control its distribution. This model offers a provocative alternative to the pharmaceuticalization of health care.

In light of ongoing revelations that FDA approval is, in itself, no assurance of pharmaceutical safety (Lyons, 2005), federal prohibitions on "one of the least physiologically toxic of psychoactive drugs" (Grinspoon, 1994: 386) seem increasingly unreasonable. In addition, reductions and restrictions in public health care programs, rising costs in corporate health care provision, and the growing ranks of the uninsured, make not-for-profit, grassroots innovations in health care all the more interesting and important. While the cost of prescription drugs have risen sharply over the past decade (Frosh, 2004), increasing numbers of Americans (now more than one-third of all U.S. adults) are making use of complementary and alternative medicines, including herbal medicines (CDC, 2004). Furthermore, the overwhelming popular support given to medical marijuana laws in eleven states across the country strongly suggests that the public is well ahead of the federal government in accepting cannabis as a promising therapeutic substance.

In short, both individual citizens and organized collectives, like WAMM, are demanding new approaches–and reviving old ones–to provide relief that is otherwise unavailable or unaffordable. WAMM's development of non-smokable alternative delivery systems for medical marijuana use provides an informative example of the way grassroots innovation and collective organization can challenge institutionalized assumptions about medicine, health care, and the alleviation of suffering.

## NOTES

1. Lyle Craker (director of the Medicinal Plant Program at the University of Massachusetts-Amherst), Rick Doblin (president of the Multidisciplinary Association for Psychedelic Studies), and Valerie Corral (co-founder of WAMM), are currently suing the U.S. federal government for obstructing medical marijuana research, including research into a way to deliver marijuana without smoking through use of a vaporizer (AP, 2004).

2. The organization's name reflects the mixed gender composition of the membership; the name was selected by co-founder Valerie Corral as an intentional feminist re-working of the more conventional use of "Man" as the universal. Here, the word "Wo/Men" represents both genders by literally including both women and men.

3. With the exception of the federally controlled marijuana garden operated by the National Institute on Drug Abuse at the University of Mississippi. On June 6, 2005, however, the Supreme Court overturned the lower court's decision; WAMM's injunction was lifted several months later. As a result, the organization decided against planting a collective garden this year.

4. Voluntary cash donations from members are accepted, but not required.

5. This is dark humor indeed as it is unusual for a month to pass without the loss of a member or two; over 150 members have died since 1996.

6. Marinol is a synthetic form of THC available in pill or suppository form by prescription.

7. The classic discussion of learning how to be a marijuana user is found in Becker (1953).

8. The same method is used to process the bud trimmings, or "shake." The resulting *kif*, however, is considerably more potent due the higher THC content found in the buds. It is used to produce higher strength medicinal products for patients suffering from the most severe pain and muscular spasms.

## REFERENCES

Associated Press. 2004. "Scientists Say Marijuana Research Blocked." Miami Herald. July 20. http://www.herald.com

Becker, Howard. 1953. "Becoming a Marihuana User." American Journal of Sociology, LIX. November: 235-42.

Center for Disease Control. 2004. "More Than One-Third of U.S. Adults Use Complementary and Alternative Medicine, According to New Governmental Survey." National Center for Health Statistics. May 27. http://www.cdc.gov/nchs/pressroom/04news/adultsmedicine.htm

Congressional Hearings by the House Committee on Governmental Reform: Subcommittee on Criminal Justice, Drug Policy, and Human Resources. 2004. Transcript of Hearings on Medical Marijuana. April 1. http://www.mapinc.org/newscmc/v04/n533/a05.html

Elders, Joycelyn. 2004. "The Myths About Medical Marijuana." Providence Journal. March 26. http://www.projo.com.

Frosh, Dan. 2004. "Drug Store Cowboys." Alternet. November 16. http://www.alternet.org/story/20512.

Grinspoon, Lester. 2000. "Whither Medical Marijuana." in Contemporary Drug Problems, vol. 27, #1. Spring 2000.

Grinspoon, Lester. 1994. *Marijuana Reconsidered.* Oakland, CA: Quick American Archives. (Reprint, with new introduction, of the 1977 Harvard University Press second edition).

Guterman, Lila. 2000. "The Dope on Medical Marijuana." Chronicle of Higher Education. June 2. http://chronicle.com.

Institute of Medicine. 1999. "Marijuana and Medicine: Assessing the Science Base." Washington DC: National Academy Press.

Kuhn, Cynthia, Scott Swartzwelder, and Wilkie Wilson. 2003. *Buzzed.* New York: Norton and Company.

Lyons, Julie S. 2005. "More pangs of doubt." San Jose Mercury News. February 15.

O'Reilly Factor. 2004. Transcript of "Are We Getting Close to Legalizing Pot?" July 7. http://www.foxnews.com

Randall, R.C. 1991. *Marijuana and AIDS.* Washington DC: Galen Press.

Randall, R.C. (Ed). 1989. *Marijuana, Medicine and the Law*; vol. 2. Washington DC: Galen Press.

Russo, Ethan. 2002. "Chronic Cannabis Use in the Compassionate Investigational New Drug Program." Journal of Cannabis Therapeutics, vol. 2 (1).

Zimmer, Lynn, and John Morgan. 1997. *Marijuana Myths, Marijuana Facts.* New York: Lindesmith Center.

# Index

In this index, page numbers in *italics* designate figures; page numbers followed by the letter "t" designate tables; *See also* cross-references designate related topics or more detailed subtopic lists.

# BOOK ORDER FORM!

Order a copy of this book with this form or online at:
http://www.haworthpress.com/store/product.asp?sku= 5787

## The Cultural/Subcultural Contexts of Marijuana Use at the Turn of the Twenty-First Century

___ in softbound at $29.95 ISBN-13: 978-0-7890-3204-1 / ISBN-10: 0-7890-3204-X.

___ in hardbound at $49.95 ISBN-13: 978-0-7890-3203-4 / ISBN-10: 0-7890-3203-1.

**COST OF BOOKS** _____

**POSTAGE & HANDLING** _____
US: $4.00 for first book & $1.50
for each additional book
Outside US: $5.00 for first book
& $2.00 for each additional book.

**SUBTOTAL** _____

In Canada: add 7% GST. _____

**STATE TAX** _____
CA, IL, IN, MN, NJ, NY, OH, PA & SD residents
please add appropriate local sales tax.

**FINAL TOTAL** _____

If paying in Canadian funds, convert
using the current exchange rate,
UNESCO coupons welcome.

❑ **BILL ME LATER:**
Bill-me option is good on US/Canada/
Mexico orders only; not good to jobbers,
wholesalers, or subscription agencies.

❑ **Signature** _____

**Payment Enclosed: $** _____

❑ **PLEASE CHARGE TO MY CREDIT CARD:**

❑ Visa ❑ MasterCard ❑ AmEx ❑ Discover
❑ Diner's Club ❑ Eurocard ❑ JCB

**Account #** _____

**Exp Date** _____

**Signature** _____
(Prices in US dollars and subject to change without notice.)

| PLEASE PRINT ALL INFORMATION OR ATTACH YOUR BUSINESS CARD |
|---|
| Name |
| Address |
| City          State/Province          Zip/Postal Code |
| Country |
| Tel          Fax |

May we use your e-mail address for confirmations and other types of information? ❑ Yes ❑ No We appreciate receiving
your e-mail address. Haworth would like to e-mail special discount offers to you, as a preferred customer.
**We will never share, rent, or exchange your e-mail address.** We regard such actions as an invasion of your privacy.

Order from your **local bookstore** or directly from
**The Haworth Press, Inc.** 10 Alice Street, Binghamton, New York 13904-1580 • USA
Call our toll-free number (1-800-429-6784) / Outside US/Canada: (607) 722-5857
Fax: 1-800-895-0582 / Outside US/Canada: (607) 771-0012
E-mail your order to us: orders@haworthpress.com

**For orders outside US and Canada,** you may wish to order through your local
sales representative, distributor, or bookseller.
For information, see http://haworthpress.com/distributors

(Discounts are available for individual orders in US and Canada only, not booksellers/distributors.)

**Please photocopy this form for your personal use.**
www.HaworthPress.com

BOF06